The Sporting Horse

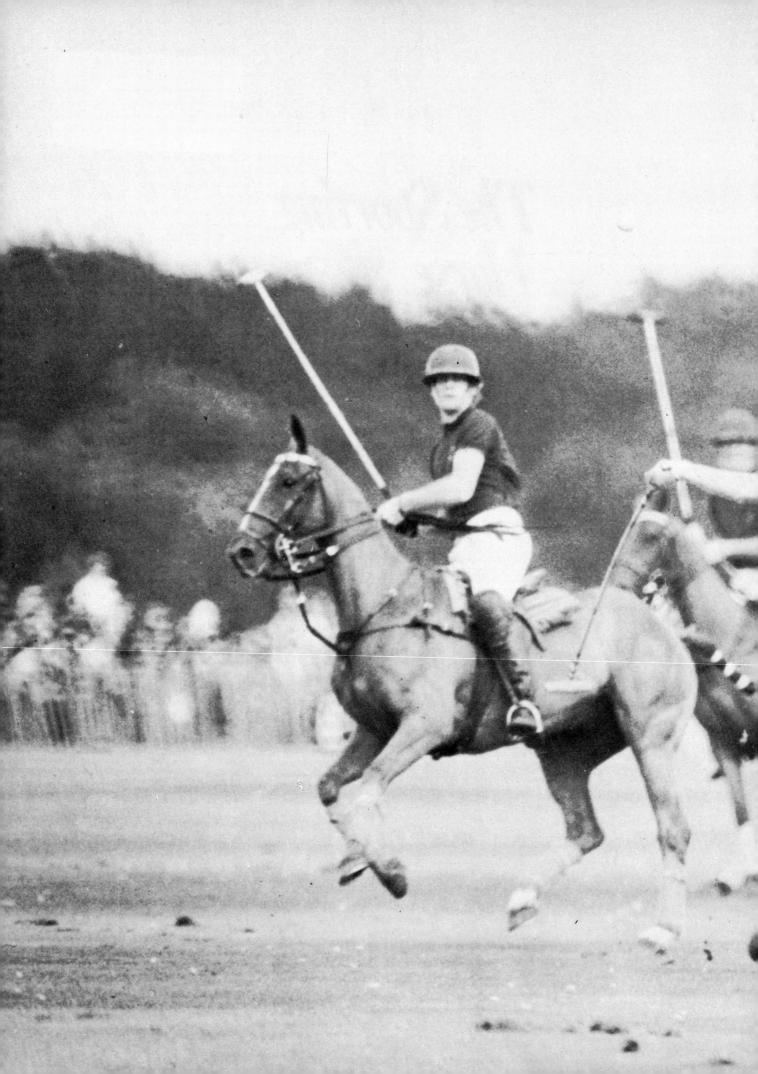

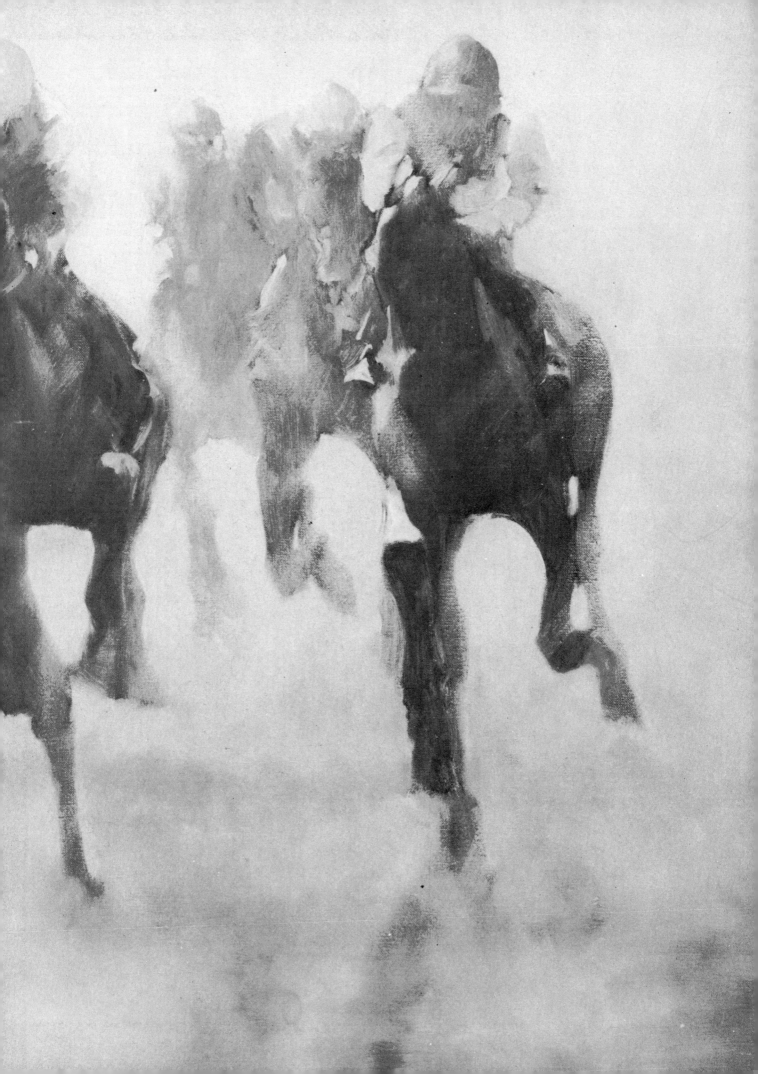

The Sporting Horse

Peter Churchill

Marshall Cavendish London & New York

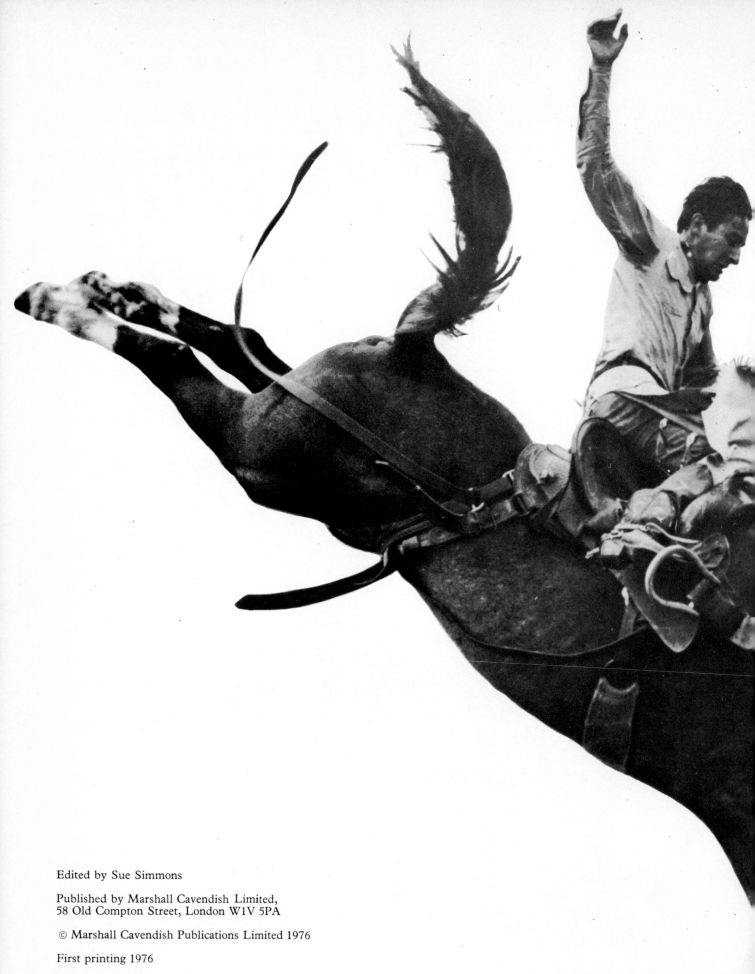

Edited by Sue Simmons

Published by Marshall Cavendish Limited,
58 Old Compton Street, London W1V 5PA

© Marshall Cavendish Publications Limited 1976

First printing 1976

ISBN 0 85685 139 6

Printed in Great Britain by Severn Valley Press Ltd

Introduction

In the twentieth century there has been a rise in the popularity of all sporting events – not least those sports involving the horse. Its traditional roles have been superseded to a great extent by machines; its usefulness now is measured in its beauty and its entertainment value to man in his increased leisure hours – for riding, competing in equestrian events or spectating.

The Sporting Horse traces the rise in these sports from the days when racing was dominated by the nobility and dressage was the preserve of the military, to the modern day when the former tasks of the horse are being turned into spectator sports.

All the great names are included. Jockeys from the amazingly successful Fred Archer to Lester Piggott, National Hunt champions of the calibre of Fred Winter and Josh Gifford, showjumping experts such as David Broome, Harvey Smith and Hartwig Steenken and the masters of precision in the dressage ring, Josef Neckermann and Lorna Johnstone.

And the great horses – flat racers from Eclipse to the recent outstanding American champion Speculator; the memorable steeplechasers such as Devon Loch, Arkle and Red Rum; showjumpers Nizefela and The Rock to the young horses now taking the honours and the horses from the latest sport to capture the public's imagination – the three-day event.

If you are interested in any aspect of the horse in sport, *The Sporting Horse* gives you a fully illustrated account of all you want to know about the rules, the history and the present-day champions of the horse world.

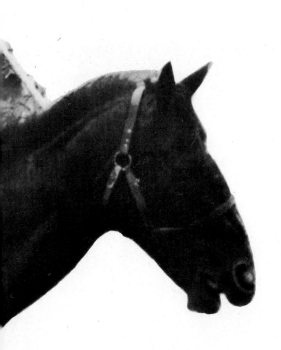

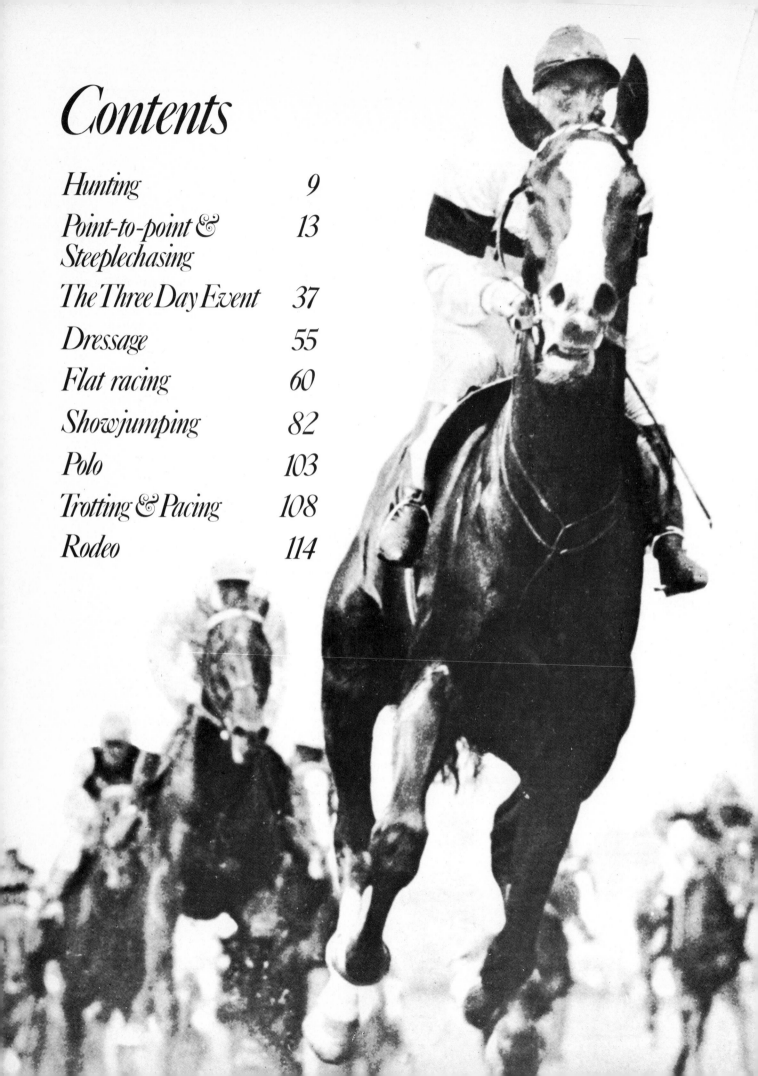

Contents

The Sporting Horse

The twentieth century has brought a greater upsurge and interest in equestrian activities than any other period in the long and complex history of the horse. In this jet-age, space-conqueroring era of ours the ancient man of war and one time beast of burden has inspired some of the most popular and exciting national sports throughout the world. Thousands of people, young and old, ride for pleasure at the weekends in England, America, Australia, Ireland and throughout Western Europe.

More and more horses are registered for show-jumping and racing every year; nearly ten thousand jumpers are recorded with the British Show Jumping Association alone. In many countries the national economy is subsidized by the revenue from Tote Betting systems on horse-racing and trotting. Equine Research Centres are part and parcel of agricultural policy in nearly every major country in the world. The horse, once thought to be obsolete with the dawning of the mechanical age, is now an important factor in the leisure of man.

Flat-racing and steeplechasing are the biggest and most popular sports of all, not only for the thrill of gambling. Like film stars, successful and well-known horses draw huge crowds to the track just to see them run. Jockeys and trainers are public figures and racegoers have their favourites in each country. From the days of 'matches' for wagers to modern times, fortunes have been made and lost on the race-track. The sport of kings is the world of the tipster, the con-man, the social climber and the small man just about to make it big. Racehorses worth millions are cosseted by devoted stable staff. And colts and fillies from humble origins, bought at bargain prices, can overnight make an unfashionable breeding-line the most valuable property on the market.

With the advancement of the mass-media, richly prized races have become major international occasions, viewed by millions of people.

Steeplechasing, always thought to be the poor relation of the racing game, has made tremendous strides since the young bloods hared from steeple to steeple. Yet many stars of National Hunt racing still have their origins in the hunting field, which continues to be a popular and well-supported sport in many parts of the globe.

Not far behind the heels of racing in popularity is international show-jumping. This relatively young sport has produced new stars that the public will flock to see. From the early days of the village-green 'Gymkhana', supported by a few military enthusiasts and sporting dealers, this equestrian spectacle has grown to unbelievable proportions. At the Royal International Horse Show, Wembley, England, a favourite venue on the world circuit, no fewer than sixty million television viewers watch the weeks jumping performed by some of the sport's top exponents.

In recent years, mainly through the ever-increasing interest in the Olympic Games, even some of the minority-interest sports, such as three-day eventing, have enlarged their more specialist following. This is one of the most complete tests the horse has to face, with a dressage test, endurance test, steeplechase, cross-country and show-jumping phases to be completed in the space of three days. The fitness and courage of both horse and rider are therefore of paramount importance in this most exacting of equestrian sports.

And polo is no longer the pastime of a few mad Englishmen galloping around in the mid-day sun, as in the days of the Raj. The sport now has its own international circuit, with national teams travelling between Argentina, the United States, Great Britain and France. Ponies scientifically bred for the job, can be worth almost as much as the fastest racehorse.

Just as hunting was the father of steeplechasing, the cowman riding the range inspired America's number one spectator sport. Rodeo or bronc-riding is the game of the American rough-rider. The rules and technicalities have become more complicated but the goal is still the simplest ever invented in equestrianism: to stay on and calm the wild, spirited horse of the great outdoors.

On the Continent and the United States, trotting racing draws the public through the turnstiles as chariot racing did in Roman times. The glamorous world of horse-racing is reflected on the tight cinder-and-tan tracks and floodlit arenas of this tough and exciting sport.

Throughout the world, people are now enjoying the pleasure the horse can give, not only by spectator sports but by participating themselves. No longer must the horse be asked to charge headlong into the enemy rank and file or to laboriously draw the plough through the fields. Yet neither will he be rendered obsolete—the developments of the 20th century have ensured him a prominent and secure place in the leisure hours of man.

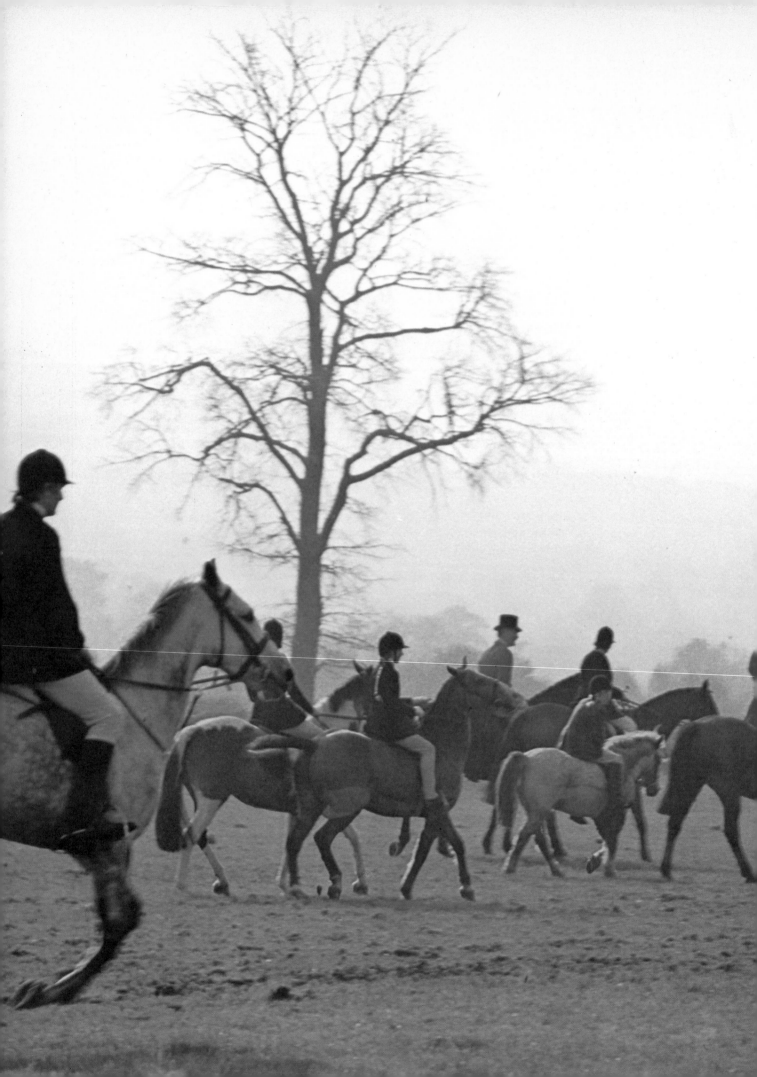

Hunting–
'..the image of war without its guilt..'

The barbarians who created Europe from the ruins of the Roman Empire were keen huntsmen. The kings and nobles of the regions that are now France and Germany not only hunted wolf, boar and stag, but also the bear, bison and the wild ox. Indeed, the prowess of rider and horse were often indications of social esteem and regard and this prowess was best demonstrated in the com-

The thin winter sunlight silhouettes the riders as young and old alike set out in search of quarry.

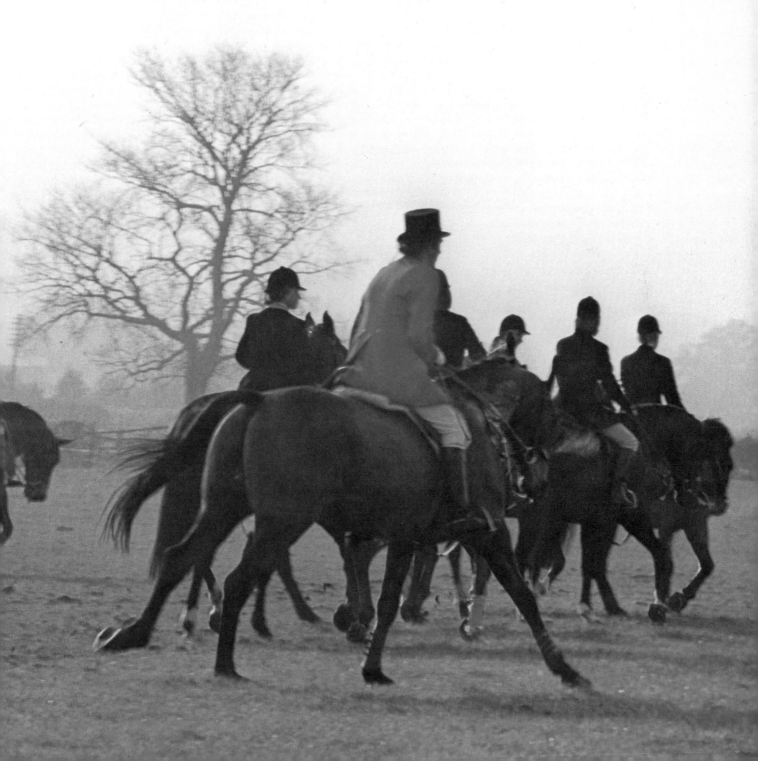

Right *The hounds move in for the kill. As with all blood sports, hunting remains a controversial issue although it has increased considerably in popularity since the Second World War.*

Below right *Staghounds alert and ready for the hunt on Exmoor where some of the finest stag hunting in England can be found. While in France hunting takes place in the forests, in England the deer must be driven out onto open moorland by the 'tufter' hounds before the rest of the hunt can join in.*

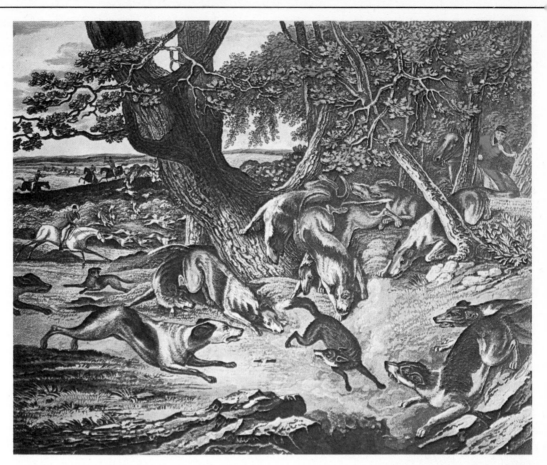

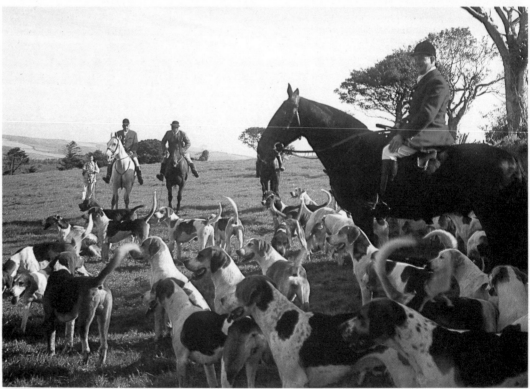

petitiveness of a chase.

By the 15th century, many books and papers had been published on the art of hunting. In 1512, the Duke of Northumberland had 15 horses in his private stable in London. Although breeds as such had not yet arrived, it is reported that he had light horses for the ladies, big trotting horses for his carriage and strong, active horses for hunting.

Hunting in the modern world

Hunting is still a major sport throughout the

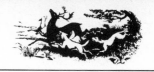

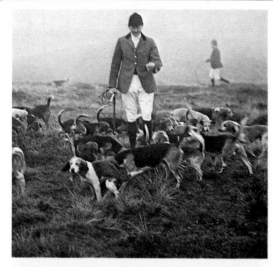

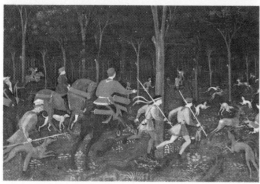

modern world. In England and Wales, there are nearly 200 packs, the majority of which hunt the fox. Most of these go hunting on average three or four times a week. The season runs from November through to the following April with stag-, deer-, and hare-hunting following more or less the same pattern.

The best horses for hunting are bred in Ireland. Its climate and the mineral-content of its land provide ideal conditions for the breeding of horses. Each year, around the second week in August, buyers from all over the world travel to the Dublin Horse Show. Besides being a shop-window for breeders, the Show is also a market-place for young hunter stock.

Fox hunting is also practised in a number of regions in America, and some of the sport's most famous packs of hounds are found in Virginia and Kentucky. The etiquette, style of dress and type of riding-country are similar to those found in England.

The effects of enclosure

Yet, it was not until the coming of the Enclosure Acts, which took several years to put into practice and eventually culminated with a final act in the late 18th century, that hunting became a more organized sport. As a result landowners and farmers were made to define their properties and fields by planting hedges or by building fences. Before this, tenant-farmers had worked strips of land and shared the common rights of grazing land, the whole being the property of one land-owner. The advent of fencing was to have an important effect on hunting and the type of horse used for the sport.

With the defining of farms came the clarification of hunting country boundaries. And the formation of famous packs like the Quorn, Beaufort, Cottesmore and the Heythrop became part of the hunting-man's folk-lore, along with exaggerated characters like John Peel, Hugo Meynell and the vivacious 19th century huntswoman Elizabeth, Empress of Austria. The dashing Captain 'Bay' Middleton of the 12th Lancers piloted the courageous Empress over the 'country' when she hunted with the fashionable packs of England. She is remembered for her remark to Bay: 'I don't mind the falls, but, remember, I will not scratch my face.' Hugo Meynell (1735–1808) was the first Master of the Quorn. He was known as the 'Hunting Jupiter' and looked upon his horses as machines that enabled him to keep company with his hounds.

In England, the Midlands became the best country for all hunting men to ride over. It was grass country, galloping country and, after the 'enclosure', a country that required the best quality, the fastest and bravest hunters, capable of jumping large fences.

Etiquette and organisation

The science of killing foxes and stags also took on a more organized form with its own strictly defined hierarchy. The Master is responsible for organizing the Hunt establishment and the 'field'. The Huntsman is the man who actually hunts the hounds and 'breaks in' the young entry (the young hounds).

In some Hunts the post of Kennel-huntsman is filled by a professional; in others the work of caring for hounds is carried out by the Master himself. Then comes the first Whipper-in, who, again, could fill the role of huntsman; his job is to help the huntsman control the pack of hounds. The second Whipper-in carries out the same function and is responsible to the huntsman. The Field Master, a member of the Hunt Committee, is a kind of 'back-up' to the Master. As his title suggests, he is responsible for the organization of the 'field'. The Hunt and its country is run by a committee, of which the Master is a member. The committee arranges finance, handles any claims for damage caused by the Hunt, sees to repairs to fencing and helps the Master in finding the money to run the pack and provide horses for the Hunt staff.

But hunting is a game besides being a sport. A game that for its players can become a real passion. It is not enough to be an excellent horse-man capable of riding through forest and open country, negotiating differing obstacles: sometimes a wall, sometimes a hedge, sometimes a gate or stream, each demanding the maximum courage of the rider and his horse. It is also a sport that demands of its followers an expert knowledge of country lore and rural life.

Left Men and hounds gather on a misty morning for a day's sport.

Below left The stag hunt is given an almost fairy-tale atmosphere in this detail from a 15th century painting by Italian artist Paolo Uccello.

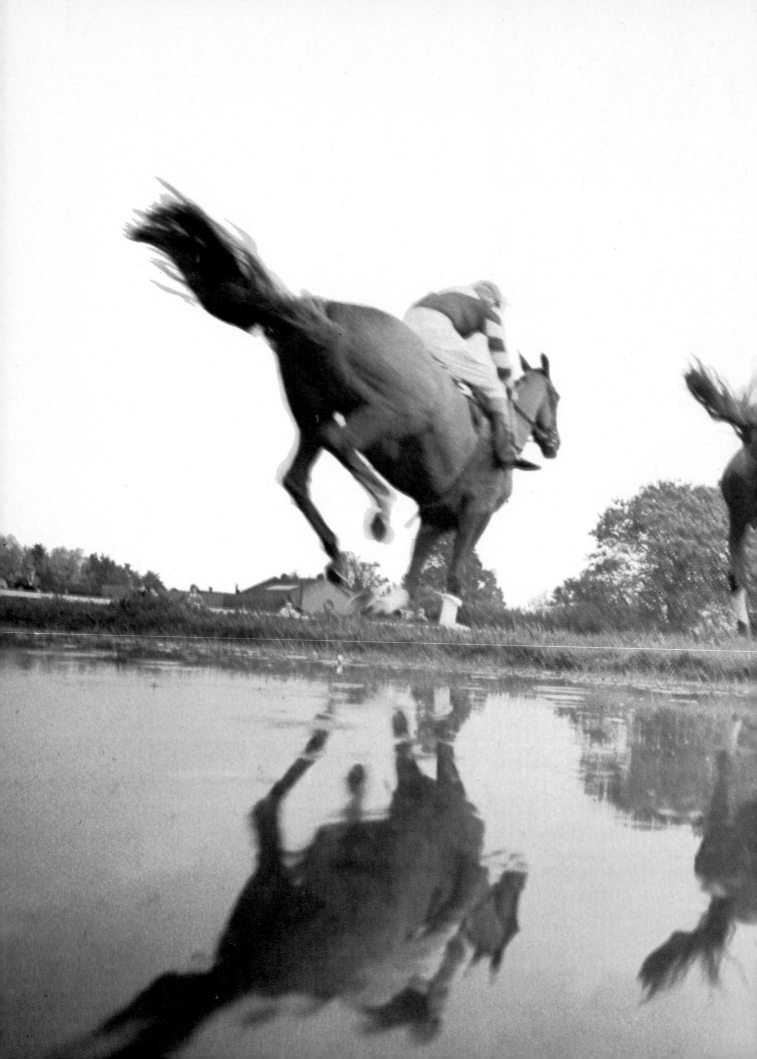

Point-to-point & Steeplechasing

Although hunting is not a race—there is no winner—it does bring out the competitive spirit of animal and man. So it is not surprising that the field of the chase should give birth to some form of racing and that such a form of racing should involve the jumping of fences at speed.

From steeple to steeple

In 18th century England, the favourite sport of the county gentry was to race in a wagered 'match' from one village steeple to the steeple of a neighbouring village, across country, jumping natural obstacles and enclosures. This was the early form of steeplechasing and point-to-pointing, and it quickly spread all over England. In Europe, where jumping does not form part of the chase, there are no records to show that racing in any form existed at that time.

Old manuscripts tell us of the first recorded match in 1752, run over approximately 7·2 km (4½ miles) in Ireland. The course was set from Buttevant Church to the spire of St Leger Church. We also find the first match involving more than two horses, in this case three, being held in Leicestershire in 1792.

Safely clearing the water, the jockey has no time to look back but only to think of the next fence. Steeplechasing is one of the most dangerous of equine sports with both horse and rider facing incredible risks, for unusually poor prospects of personal gain.

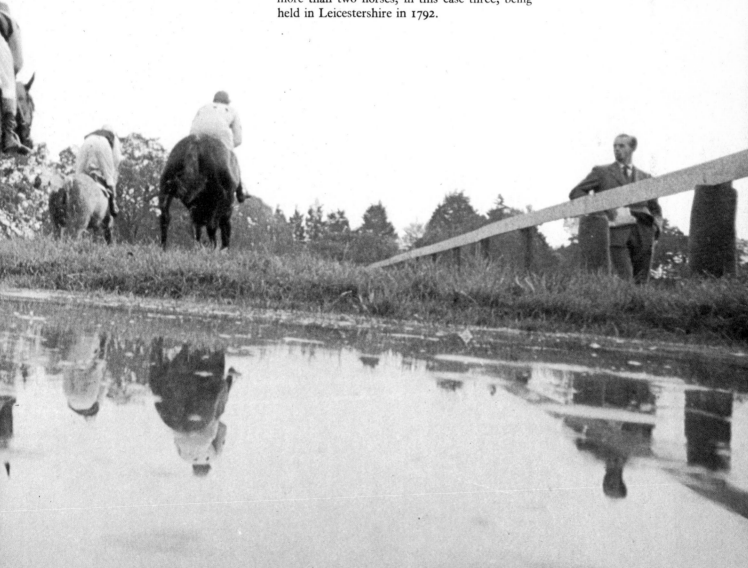

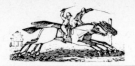

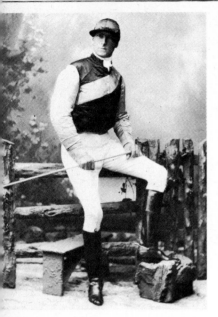

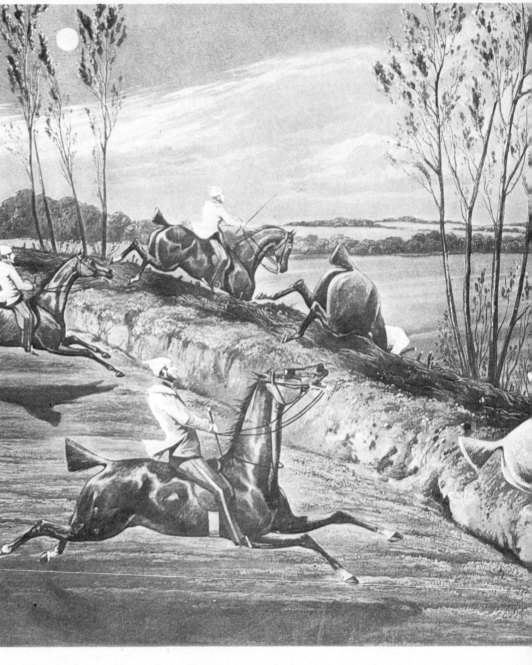

Above *An early steeple-chase jockey, Roddy Owen, complete with his long racing whip and sharp spurs.*

Right and far right *Two early prints purporting to show the first ever steeple-chase being run by moonlight in the early 1800s.*

Top right *The first Grand National with the field taking the formidable stonewall in front of the Grandstand. Lottery, the eventual winner is shown just behind the leader.*

Top far right
A contemporary artist's interpretation of Becher's famous fall.

In 1810 the first modern-style steeplechase was run over a planned course at Bedford, England. Eight fences had to be jumped over a distance of 4·8 km (3 miles) and the race was run in heats. The eventual victor was a big jumper called Fugitive.

A legend in his own lifetime

The hunting field produced one of the most famous of the early steeplechase jockeys, Dick Christian. Born in 1779 in the small village of Cottesmore, Leicestershire, one of the most famous hunting counties in England, Christian became a legend in his own lifetime. Henry Hall Dixon, a contemporary sportswriter writing under the name of 'The Druid', is on record as saying, 'Dick Christian had practically sounded the depth of every ditch and brook in Leicestershire for more than half a century: but its fox-

hunters had never half sounded him in return.'

'The best 'chaser I have ever ridden'

The sheer exuberance, excitement and danger of early English steeplechasing is portrayed in the following quaint but colourful account of a challenge between Dick Christian and one of the local squires. His portrait records not only the cunning and ingenuity of the riders but also the courage and strength of the two horses—Clinker and Clasher.

'Clinker's and Clasher's was a great match; they said it was 1500 guineas (3760 dollars) a side. They sent for me the night before, did Captain White and Captain Rose, and locked me into their room; then they gave me their orders: they says, "We mean you to wait, Dick." I said, "You'd better let me let the horse go along, gentlemen, and not upset him; he'll take a great

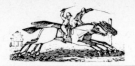

14

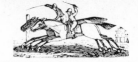

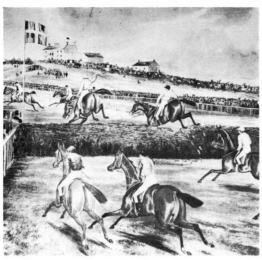

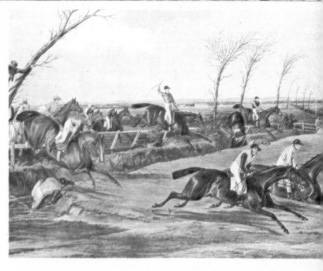

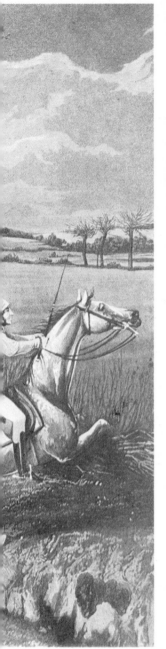

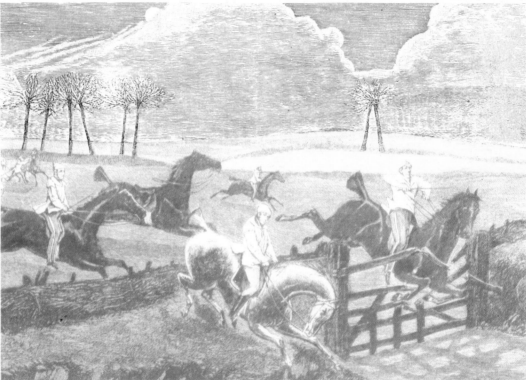

deal more out of himself by waiting.'' So I got them persuaded round.

'We weighed at Dalby, the Squire and I was never in such condition. They were walking the horses about, and Captain Rose he says to me, "Clinker looks well." I said, "He looks too well, Captain." Then he lifted me up, and he tells me the orders were changed, and I must wait. "Its giving away a certainty," says I, "and if I get a fall then I am all behind." But it was of no manner of use talking.

'Sir Vincent Cotton and Mr Gilmour, they started us, and Mr Maher he was umpire. We rode twelve stone apiece: I was in tartan, and the Squire, of course, he'd be in green. When we are at the post, he says, "Now Christian, I know what your orders are—I do ask one thing: don't jump on me if I fall." "I give you my word, Squire, I won't."

'We were almost touching each other over Sharplands, and just before the road I says, "Squire, your beat for 100 pounds," but he never made no answer. Then we met some rails; such stiff 'uns. Clasher hits them with all four legs, and chucked the Squire right on his neck; Clinker took 'em like a bird.

'We were each in a mess then; the Squire he lands in a bog, and his horse makes a dead stop, it did take a great deal out of him; then I jumps right into the dung heap, up to Clinker's knees; we had no manner of idea the things were there. Going up John O'Gaunt's field we were together, but I turns to get some rails in the corner; he was such a good one at rails was Clinker; I thought he was winning, but dreary me, down he comes at the last fence, dead beat.

'Clinker he lays for some minutes, then he gets up as lively as ever; the horse looked no

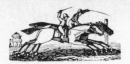

manner of form, as round as a hoop, for all the world as if he were going to Horncastle Fair. They held Clasher up, and they flung water in his face, and he won in the last hundred yards from superior training, and that's the honest truth. Many didn't like Clinker, but I never got on so good a steeplechaser.'

Many steeplechase jockeys were to make a similar remark in the future: 'The best 'chaser I have ever ridden.' This was and remains the tradition of steeplechasing, the horse is the most vital part of the sport. As brave as the rider on his back, he gives every muscle of effort, his heart and, tragically, sometimes his life.

Point-to-point

Jump-racing is like the battlefield, demanding skill, stamina, strength and sportsmanship. Those early forms of steeplechasing for wagers are today manifested in point-to-point racing where rich man, horse-dealer and farmer race against each other for no material gain but for the privilege of producing the best hunt chaser in their country. From November to February they hunt together to qualify their horses for the point-to-point races. But once qualified, and with a certificate signed by the Master stating that the horse has been fairly hunted, the rivalry to win the big race at the local track begins in earnest.

The race-card usually consists of a Member's race, confined to members of the organizing hunt. This is followed by a Maiden race, for horses that have not won a race, and an Open race, for all subscribers to bona fide hunts in England and Wales. These preceed the Adjacent Hunts race, for horses from neighbouring packs, and a Ladies' race.

The local point-to-point is usually a picnic day

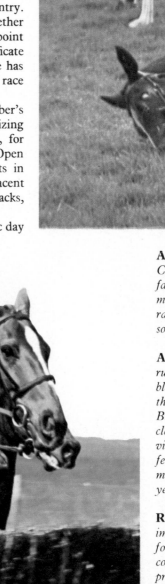

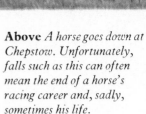

Above *A horse goes down at Chepstow. Unfortunately, falls such as this can often mean the end of a horse's racing career and, sadly, sometimes his life.*

Above right *A jockey ruefully rubs his bruised and bleeding face after a fall at the infamous Becher's Brooke, a fence which still claims a large number of victims each year. However, few jockeys are daunted and many come back to compete year after year.*

Right and left *An important schooling ground for horse and jockey, the country point-to-point also provides the opportunity for women to compete on equal terms with men.*

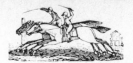

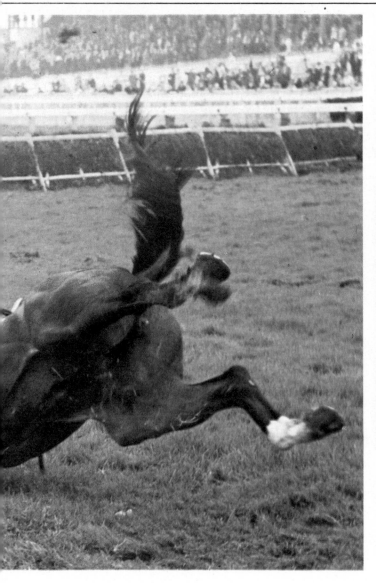

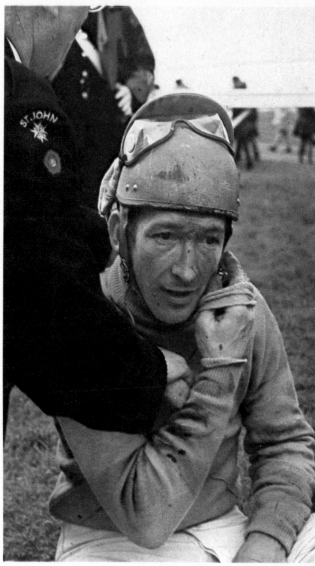

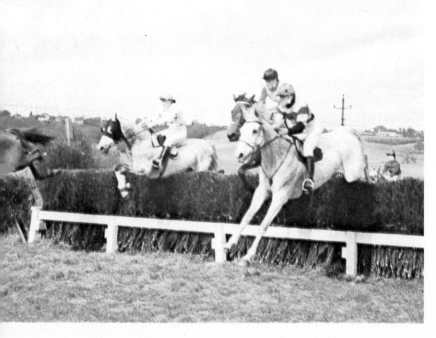

for all the families of the district. Farmers, tradesman, landowners, bookies and all the other people of the neighbourhood throng to the races to provide a colourful, lively and excited pano-rama.

This is the world of the amateur, the enthu-siast, of the open ditch jumped from three strides out. But from this amateur world has sprouted the world of professional steeplechasing. The ambitious amateur, or 'bumper', with enough money to support his hobby, dreams of taking on the big boys on the professional jumping tracks. And the amateur with little money, but with talent and hope, dreams of being spotted by a top-line trainer and being asked to turn 'pro' and ride first jockey for him.

The National Hunt Committee
By the beginning of the 19th century the Rules of Racing were set up and permanent tracks were laid out, enabling steeplechasing to become truly professional. A Mr Weatherby, publisher of the Racing Calendar, started the General Stud Book which records the linear descendancy of all British thoroughbred horses. James Weatherby,

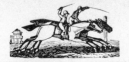

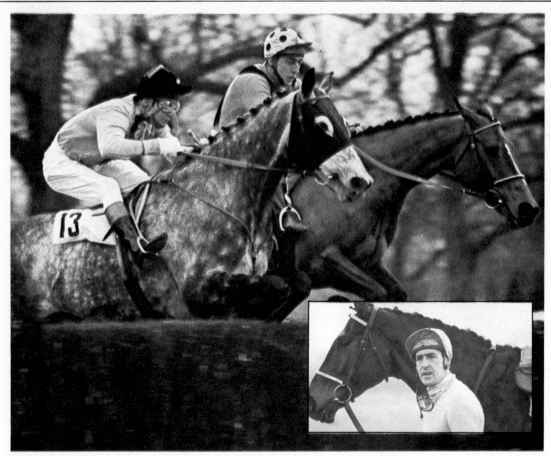

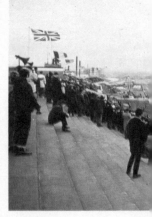

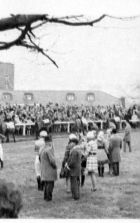

Above *Bannon's Star with Josh Gifford up leads Chaou II. Many National Hunt jockeys start their careers on the flat and like Josh Gifford turn to steeplechasing through weight problems.*

a relative, was the first Keeper of the Match Book, a record of races, weights and wagers. Although these two administrators of the Turf did not work together it was not long before the family formed what is now known as Weatherby and Sons. Weatherby and Sons are now Secretaries of the National Hunt Committee, the governing body of all steeple and hurdle-racing in the British Isles, and act as the Registry Office of both the Jockey Club and the National Hunt Committee. The Racing Calendar, owned by the Jockey Club, is published by them and is usually considered the supreme authority in British racing.

The Grand National

As the century progressed, jump-racing began to take a more organized form and in 1837 a Liverpool hotelier conceived the idea of staging a steeplechase that was to become the most famous and the most wanted prize in steeplechasing, the Grand National. Although not known then as the Grand National, and run at a place called Maghull, it was the inspiration behind the forming of a race committee, which included such sporting dignitaries as the Earls of Derby and Sefton, Lord George Bentinck and Lord Robert Grosvenor, and the course was moved to its present home at Aintree near Liverpool.

At that time the course fences consisted of a stone-wall, now replaced by the water jump, a stretch of ploughland, now turfed, to be galloped over, and the last fence was a hurdle. Apart from

the sloping take-offs and some slight modification to the thorn and spruce obstacles the track has changed very little since the February of 1839 when Jem Mason rode home his mount Lottery after making nearly all the running from a horse called Seventy Four. Behind them came a small number of stragglers, tired and beaten—all that were left of the original 17 starters.

Becher's Brook

It was in this same race that the name of Aintree's greatest sportsman was stamped on the history of the race and on the dreaded fence that became known as Becher's Brook. As Jem Mason and Lottery were coming to the stiffest fence on the course, a double rails and a large ditch dammed on the far side, they narrowly avoided collision with Conrad ridden by Captain Becher who had served with Wellington in the Peninsular War. Conrad hit the rails and Becher went straight over his head into the ditch. Hence the name Becher's Brook. But it was not the end of steeplechasing's greatest amateur. He remounted and chased after Lottery. After nearly a mile he caught up with the leader only to part company from Conrad again at another fence.

This is the first of many stories and legends of Liverpool that make the magic, the glory and the fascination of what we now call the Grand National, the greatest steeplechase in the world. Huge fields, sometimes numbering up to 50 and over, and the hazards of the difficult fences have caused numerous injuries and some deaths. At

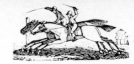

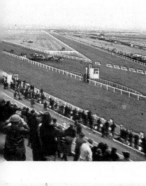

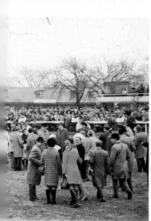

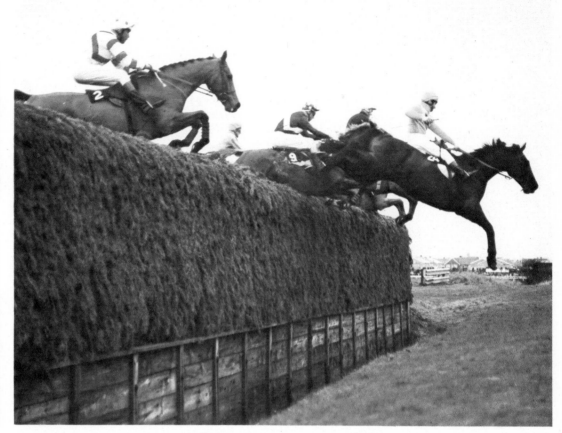

one time there was an outcry that it should be banned. But each year it produced plenty of spirit and great steeplechasing.

Aintree

Aintree racecourse is situated on a spacious triangular expanse of green turf, just outside Liverpool, and nowadays surrounded by industrial development. The huge old Grandstands, described by many visitors as antiquated and neglected, have a majesty and aura of their own. Standing alone on the well-worn terraces in the early morning mist, one can almost hear the cheering crowds of days gone by shouting home the legendary heroes of the National: Adb El Kader, the first dual winner in 1850 and 1851; George Stevens, the great jump-jockey who was the first Aintree specialist, winning no less than five Grand Nationals including a double on the Colonel in 1869 and 1870. (Stevens was eventually killed tragically in 1871, whilst out riding near his home after his retirement from steeplechasing).

Charles Kinsky, an Austrian prince, became one of the small band of owner-riders to win the Grand National with his mare Zoedone in 1883. Those phantom crowds would have seen Ernie Piggott, grandfather of crack flat-race rider Lester Piggott, coming home on Jerry M in 1912. He followed this with a double victory (one at the wartime substitute track at Gatwick in Sussex) on one of the greatest steeplechasers of the era, Poethlyn.

The toughest course in the world

The course starts its 7·2km (4 miles 856 yards) journey to the right of the sprawling stands near the Sefton Yard Stables. The long run to the first of the 30 fences is often similar to a cavalry charge, as jockeys manoeuvre for position, trying to find a good 'berth' for the galloping steed beneath them.

The first two fences are made of plain thorn and spruce, standing at 1·37m (4ft 6in) and 1·4m (4ft 7in). The third is the first of Liverpool's gaping 1·83m (6ft) open ditches with a 1·52m (5ft) fence. At the side of the ditch is a politely-placed white picket gate for the fallers to walk out of the ditch. The horses then race on to two more plain obstacles before the jockeys' hearts start thumping and the adrenaline starts flowing at the sight of the most famous fence in the world, Becher's Brook. A 1·47m (4ft 10in) fence with a 1·67m (5ft 6in) brook and a drop of over 1·83m (6ft), Becher's Brook has to be taken at racing speed. A number of horses usually fall.

The survivors then race on the lush turf, the race-strip dog-legs to a 1·22m (4ft) fence, placed at a slight angle. Here the experienced Aintree jockey looks for his line to the Canal Turn. This must be approached correctly for, on landing, horse and rider have a near 90-degree turn to make for the run to Valentine's Brook. Once over the 1·52m (5ft) dark green thorn mound and 1·67m (5ft 6in) brook, it is a straight run to fences 10, 11 (the second of the formidable open ditches) and 12, another 'five-footer' (1·52m)

Above *The leaders take the most daunting fence of the course – Becher's Brook. A 4ft. 10in. (1·47m) fence with a drop of over 6ft. (1·83m), it has to be taken at racing speed.*

Centre *Two scenes from Aintree, the home of the Grand National. Often criticised for its neglected appearance, the course holds a majesty and aura of its own for the enthusiast.*
Above *A view from the Grandstand past which the jockey must ride twice before finishing the arduous course.*
Below *The paddock just before the start of the most famous steeplechase in the world.*

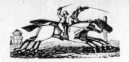

followed by a ditch. Any survivors now start the long gallop past the Anchor Bridge over the Melling Road, and round the sweeping turn to fences 13 and 14. Next time round, these will be the second-to-last and last jumps for the lucky jockeys and horses.

The crowd in the stands can see the runners clearly as they race in front of them to the 15th fence, the third of the open ditches, known as The Chair. The riders can see the winning-post, but on this circuit it is of no importance, for

instead there is the water-jump coming up very quickly. Fronted with a small 0·6m (2ft) hedge, the shimmering water stretches 3·66m (12ft). This water jump is not sloped on the landing-side, so if any foot is misplaced jockey and horse are liable to fall in a rain of pounding hooves and jockey's shouts. The dreams of owner and trainer, breeder, gambler and even the stable hands, also fall.

The battle is not yet won, for man and horse must dig deeper into their reserves of courage

Right *The National course is roughly triangular in shape. Each year four fences are rebuilt, each new fence taking thirty lorry loads of thorn and approximately six weeks for completion.*

Below *In the confusion of landing, the 1971 winner, Specify, in the green and purple colours, struggles to maintain his feet and position.*

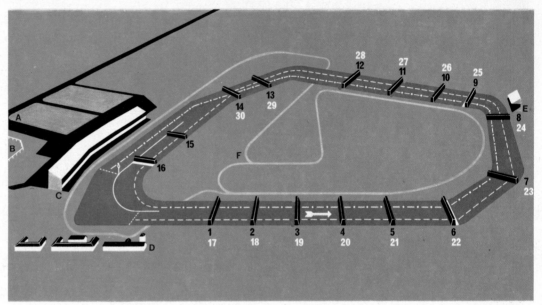

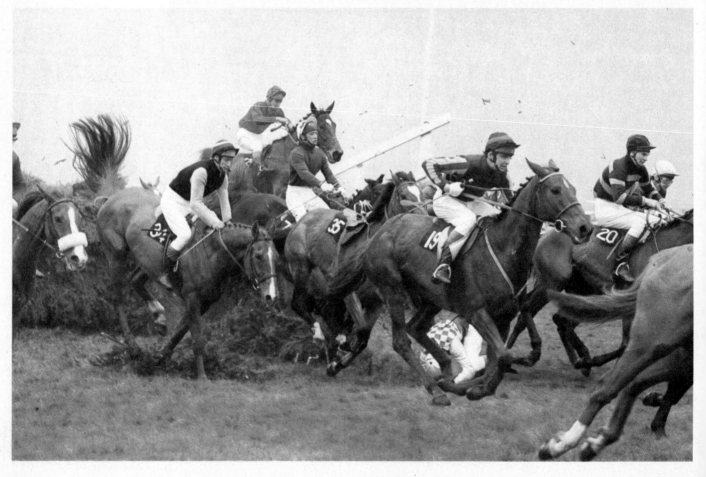

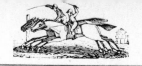

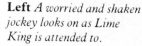

and stamina to turn out into the country once again and face the demanding Becher's Brook, the Canal and Valentine's for a second and deciding circuit.

Such is the gruelling stage of the Grand National on which both jockey and horse not only give a skilful and polished performance but also every ounce of cunning, stamina and sense of tactics they possess.

The first American challenge

In 1928, 42 horses and jockeys lined up for a Grand National which was to become legendary. Two American horses challenged for the first time. These were Billy Barton, which had won over $40,000 (£16,736) on the flat and took the American Grand National, the Maryland Hunt Cup, the Virginia Gold Cup and many other important American steeplechases, and Burgowright, also a winner of the Maryland Hunt Cup.

Easter Hero, an English horse owned by an American, turned this race into a sensation. Coming into the Canal Turn, he misjudged his approach and was straddled across the top of the fence. The sight of this unfortunate horse on top of the fence frightened many of the other horses. And among many who refused at it were Burgowright and his American jockey 'Downey' Bonsal. Billy Barton, ridden by the English professional Tom Culliman, set the pace for the remainder but going into the last, with only two left standing, the American horse fell, to leave amateur

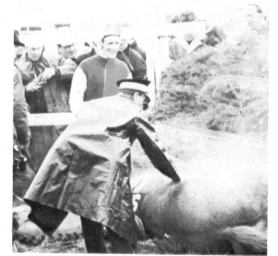

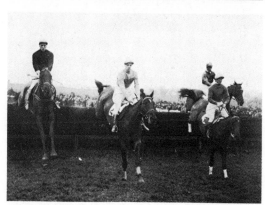

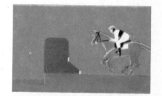

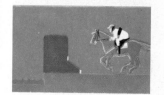

Left *A worried and shaken jockey looks on as Lime King is attended to.*

Below left *The great Golden Miller lands safely to take the 1936 Cheltenham Gold Cup.*

Below *A profile of two of the Grand National fences, the Chair and Valentine's Brook.*

Bottom *Falling horses and riders cause grave problems for the pursuing riders.*

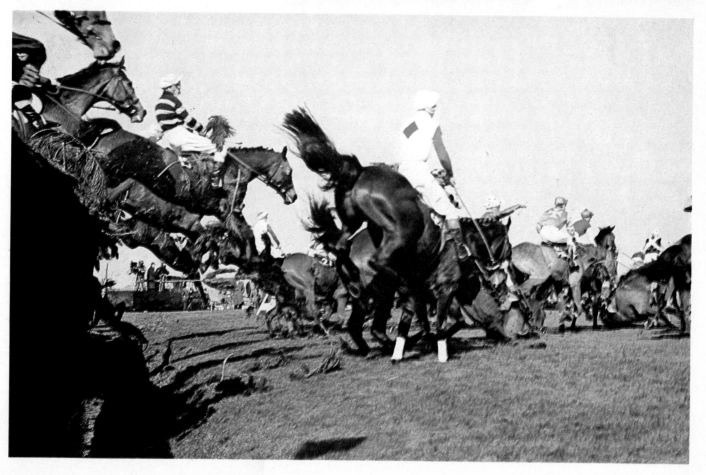

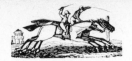

Right *Lord Anthony Mildmay on Cromwell, the horse on which he so nearly achieved his life's ambition in 1948 of winning the National. In 1936 he had also been robbed of almost certain victory riding Davy Jones when his rein broke, allowing the horse to run out at the very last fence.*

Below *1935 and 1936 were the years of the great Reynoldstown who took the Grand National in both years.*

Below right *The great steeplechaser, Golden Miller. During the 1930s he took the Cheltenham Gold Cup on five successive occasions. He, however, did not have the same success in the Grand National. But in 1934 he managed to complete the double, a still unbeaten record, by taking the Cheltenham Gold Cup and the Grand National in the same year.*

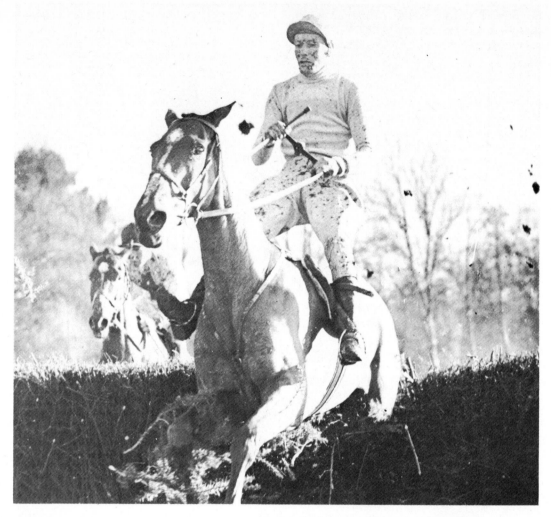

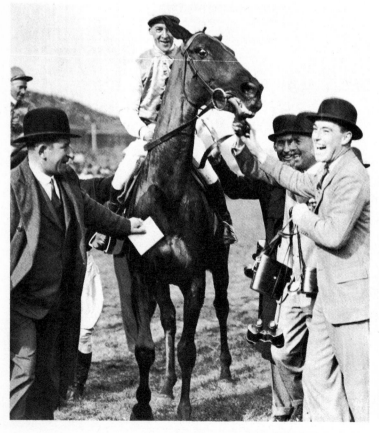

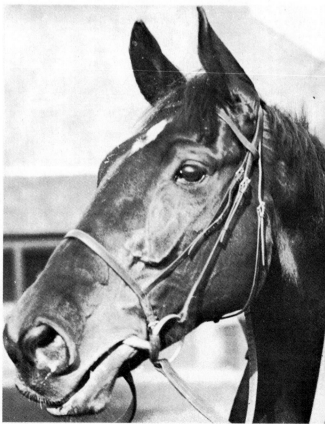

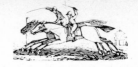

rider Bill Dutton and his mount Tipperary Tim with the race at their mercy. Culliman eventually remounted Billy Barton to finish second. Tipperary Tim, returned at 100 to 1, had changed hands as a yearling for a mere 50 guineas ($125).

Golden Miller

The Grand National, the toughest course in the world, was conquered in the record time of 9min 20·4s by what many claim to have been the greatest steeplechaser of all time, the Honorable Dorothy Paget's Golden Miller. Winner of four successive Cheltenham Gold Cups, the last one achieved after his 1934 win at Aintree, this horse of the century was bred from an ex-hunting mare, Miller's Pride, by an Irish five guinea stallion called Goldcourt.

Gerry Wilson, the jockey most closely-identified with this exceptional horse, rode him in this fastest-yet Grand National. Golden Miller swept all before him, winning nearly all the important steeplechases of his time. But the 1934 Grand National was the crowning glory of his brilliant career and the proudest moment for his eccentric owner Dorothy Paget. Miss Paget was a millionairess, plump and plain-faced, an incurable gambler and an extremely difficult woman to work for. It is said she changed her trainers and jockeys more often than a head-waiter changes his table-napkins.

But for all her peculiarities, this woman became a great patron of horse racing and her adored horse, Golden Miller, was the first real equine star, as popular in his day as the Hollywood star was in his.

'There was never a harder rider . . .'

Both 1935 and 1936 were the years of the great horse Reynoldstown. The second leg of his double in 1936 went into the annals of Aintree as another sensational and dramatic Grand National. Lord Anthony Bingham Mildmay, then known as Anthony Mildmay, was the most popular amateur rider of his day. At the age of 25 'Lordie', as racegoers called him, was at the head of the amateur riders' list under National Hunt Rules. In the 1936 National he was leading going into the second last fence on Davy Jones. Just as they were approaching this obstacle after four gruelling miles, the rein broke and Davy Jones suddenly lost all stamina. Reynoldstown, ridden by Fulke Walwyn, also an amateur and a man who was to become one of the all time greats as a National Hunt trainer, was able to go on and notch up his second Aintree victory.

The cruel hand of fate was to strike 'Lordie' Mildmay again. In the 1948 Grand National his horse Cromwell started favourite. The popular pair gave their backers a splendid run for their money. On the turn for home it looked as if Lordie was about to achieve his lifetime ambition and win the National, but on the long run to the last two fences and the winning post Mildmay's body suddenly seized up in pain. As legacy of a broken neck, he had a tendency to be attacked by sudden cramp and on passing the post in third place it was realized that he had ridden the courageous Cromwell almost blind, unable to lift his head in the last mile.

Lord Mildmay and Cromwell were two of the great characters of steeplechasing in the years after World War II and it was largely thanks to his enthusiasm and support that the British Royal Family, particularly Queen Elizabeth II and Queen Elizabeth the Queen Mother, were to take such a keen interest in the sport.

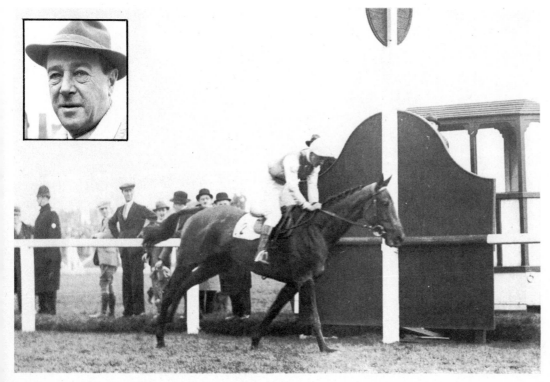

Left *Reynoldstown being ridden past the finishing post to complete the historic double by jockey now turned trainer, Fulke Walwyn, trainer of both the famous Mandarin and Mill House.*

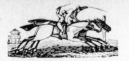

The first American winner

As Europe awaited World War II, a small American jumper crossed the Atlantic with the sole intention of being the first American to go into the winner's enclosure at the end of the 1938 Grand National. This was the American Pony, the nickname given to Mrs Marion Dupont Scott's diminutive Battleship. Winner of the American Grand National at Belmont Park, this big-hearted little horse was a son of the mighty Man o' War, a famous American thoroughbred, and was ridden at Aintree by Bruce Hobbs, the 1·9m (6ft 3in) 17-year-old son of his English trainer.

The seasoned jumping-fans did not rate their chances. Some of the mountainous fences of Aintree were higher than Battleship's 15 hands 1in frame (1·55m). By the time he jumped the last fence the crowd were on their feet shouting him home against Royal Danieli, an Irish horse. A riderless horse forced Battleship out to the far side of the run-in. The Irish horse had the favoured berth on the inside rails. Running for the line neck-and-neck, the brave little Battleship passed the post to win by the shortest of short heads. Battleship returned to Mrs Scott's Virginia estate to become one of the foundation sires of her racing stock.

In 1946, the turnstiles of Aintree clicked again after the lapse of World War II. And in the following years the record books registered great horses and jockeys such as Freebooter, whom some professionals consider the greatest steeplechaser of all time, the little mare Nickel Coin ridden by Johnny Bullock, the fantastic riding feats of Bryan Marshall, who had two wins, Pat Taaffe and others. Then, in 1956 came the tragic saga of Devon Loch.

The tragedy of Devon Loch

Her Royal Highness Queen Elizabeth, the Queen Mother, accompanied by her daughters Queen Elizabeth and Princess Margaret, watched as her gelding Devon Loch, ridden by Dick Francis, strode out of the paddock to go down to the start for what was to be the bitterest hard-luck story in the history of the race. This was not her only notable runner, for M'As-tu-vu, the mount of Arthur Freeman, was also in the line-up.

At the water, Sundew, ridden by Fred Winter, led from Eagle Lodge, ridden by Alan Oughton with E.S.B., the mount of Dave Dick, and Devon Loch in close attendance. Over Becher's Brook for the second time, champion jockey Fred Winter and Sundew (winner the following year) parted company. E.S.B. and Devon Loch then led the field. Racing to the last fence, Devon

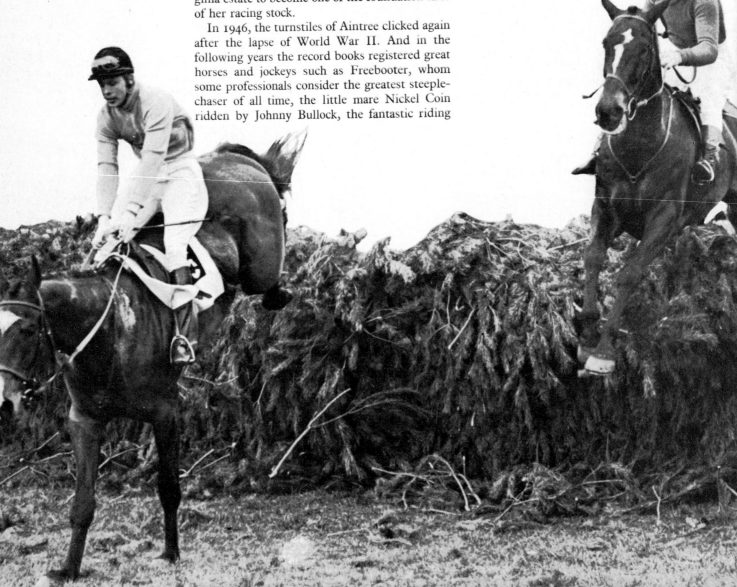

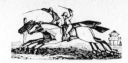

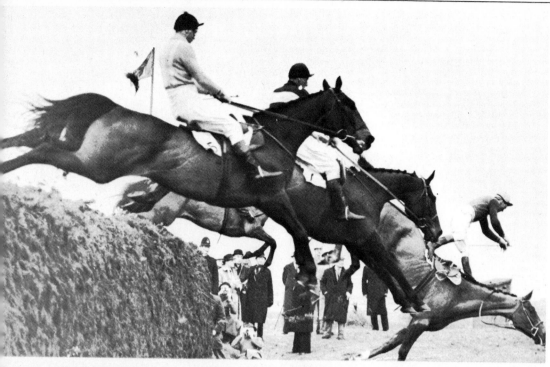

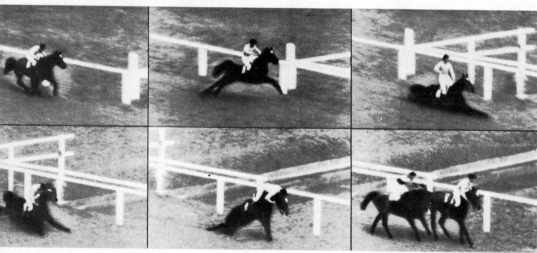

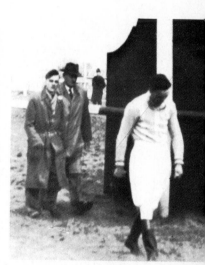

Loch was just ahead of E.S.B., and landing on the flat for the long and testing run to the line, Devon Loch had the race at his mercy. The long-legged Dave Dick accepted defeat and dropped his hands on to the neck of the tired E.S.B., allowing him to plod on at a steady but unforced pace, to a hoped-for second place.

The crowd began to realize that a first Royal victory was on the cards and they shouted with excitement. Coasting home Dick Francis waved his stick at the cheering crowd. But the unbelievable happened. As Devon Loch approached the winning-post, he cocked his ears and started to rise in the air. He sprawled and skidded on the ground, his four legs unnaturally spread-eagled on the turf. Francis was forced out on to the neck of the struggling horse. Dave Dick, seeing the Royal horse sprawled on the ground, swept by on E.S.B., to win perhaps the hollowest victory any owner has ever had in the history of the Grand National.

What happened? That is the unanswerable question still asked whenever racing-men meet and discuss such famous incidents. Did Devon Loch see an imaginary fence and attempt to jump it? Was he so exhausted that he had no control over his limbs? Or was it, as Dick Francis claims, that the roar of the crowd startled the horse and in checking himself he lost his balance and fell? The quiet, even-tempered and vice-less Devon Loch was described by Noel Murless, the great trainer of so many classic winners, as 'the clumsiest horse I have ever sat on. Even in his slower paces, he would stumble walking over a twig.' Did the Royal Devon Loch just simply trip over?

Jay Trump

The Grand National has had its share of trage-dies and melodramas. But it also had its fairy tales. Fairy-tales are rare in most walks of life but in the sport of steeplechasing fantasy can become

The unluckiest loser of all time – Devon Loch. **Top** *Clearing Becher's Brook successfully for the second time, half a length behind the eventual winner, ESB.*

Above left *The fall that cost Devon Loch the race and denied the first Royal victory.* **Above** *The disconsolate jockey, Dick Francis, leaving the field.*

Left *Jay Trump leads Freddie over the last fence of the 1965 Grand National in the first victory by an American horse ridden by an American rider.*

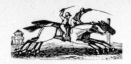

reality overnight. The story of the American jumper Jay Trump is perhaps the most well-known of fairy-tales in the history of Aintree.

Three times winner of the American timber classic, the Maryland Hunt Cup, and holder of the track-record for the 6·4km (4 miles)—a sizzling 8min 42·2 sec—Jay Trump was found by his dedicated amateur jockey, Tommy Crompton Smith, in a small yard in a shanty-town. This horse, with neither pedigree nor racing credentials, changed hands for $2000 (£836) and left the stables of Charles Town, West Virginia with Tommy Crompton Smith who as a boy dreamed of winning the Grand National. They were heading for fame and fortune on the tracks of Glyndon (Maryland), Aintree, and Auteuil (Paris) before returning to Glyndon for a last honourable triumph.

After a successful career in timber-racing, the owner and trainer of Jay Trump decided that an attempt at the Grand National was on if a good English trainer could be found. In England, one of the greatest jump-jockeys, Fred Winter, had retired from riding and started training. In his first season as a trainer the ex-champion, who rode two winners of the great race—Sundew and Kilmore—was already turning out winners with the same regularity as he rode them in the major races. Tommy Smith selected him as trainer, owner Mrs Stephenson agreed and the services of Fred Winter were engaged. Jay Trump soon settled in the vastly different atmosphere of an English racing-stable, and in his preliminary races soon qualified to run and be handicapped in the Grand National.

In 1965, the year Jay Trump was to compete, the sporting world was shocked to hear that the owner of the course, Mrs Mirabel Topham, had announced that she intended to sell the track to a property-developer. Lord Sefton, whose family connection with the course goes back to Lottery, the winner of the 1839 Grand National, stepped in and saved the race. Because of all the publicity, a record crowd turned up at the course to see what they thought would be the last Grand National.

The great Scottish horse Freddie, which came from the ranks of the hunter-chaser, was made favourite by the backers. The 47 starters spread across the 36·58m (40yd) wide cambered track to face the starting-tape, but by now this was a spectacle with a difference. The all-seeing eye of the television-camera was there for the first time to relay the race live to a large audience around the world. The American combination was about to make history, and the entire world would be there to see it. The shrewd Fred Winter gave young Tommy Smith the advice: hunt it for the first circuit, then sit down and start race-riding it.

At Valentine's Brook for the first time round, the favourite Freddie, ridden by Pat McCarron, was leading. Just behind him was Jay Trump, with Kapeno and Dave Dick between them and Leedsy, the mount of Willie Robinson, just on

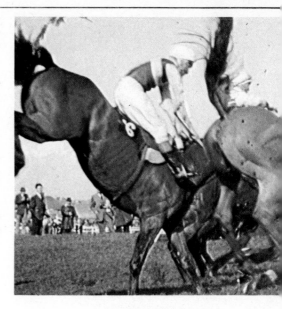

their heels. Nearly half the field swept round the sharp turn to go out in to the country for the second time. Two fences out, Freddie and Jay Trump had drawn clear and the battle was on. Going to the last, Jay Trump led Freddie by a length. Now the Scotsman and the American were locked together in a duel of champions on the long run for the post. Freddie was giving 2·27kg (5lb) to Jay Trump, and on the line the American was home and dry by three-quarters of a length.

The fairy-tale had happened. Tommy Crompton Smith became the first American rider to win the National; Jay Trump was the unexpected champion; Fred Winter had trained the winner of the Grand National, in his first season as a trainer. And Mrs Mary Stephenson from Ohio walked the hallowed path, as many owners before her had done, from racecourse to winner's enclosure. All the team connected with this great horse, down to stable hands and farrier, had made racing history. Jay Trump went on to finish a good second in the Grand Steeple de Paris and then returned to his native country to win his third Maryland Hunt Cup before retirement.

Foinavon—the rank outsider

If Jay Trump was the rags-to-riches winner, then Foinavon must rank as the loneliest victor at Aintree. He was a horse with no credentials, very little form, and ridden by an unknown jockey, Johnnie Buckingham. All the horses were still running as the group started the course the second time round. Then at the fence after Becher's Brook a riderless horse ran across the next fence, taking the fence and all but one of the field with him. Foinavon, plodding along at the back, tailed off and was not disturbed by the calamity. Johnnie Buckingham realized what had happened, steered clear of the disaster-area, jumped the fence and found himself with seven more fences and almost all the time in the world. Fence after fence, the tired Foinavon plodded on to run out the official winner by 15 lengths and a

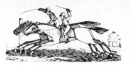

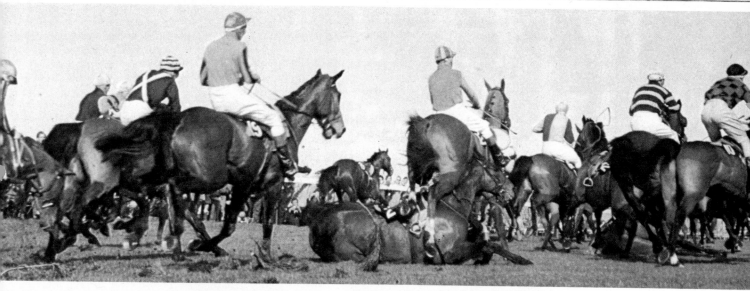

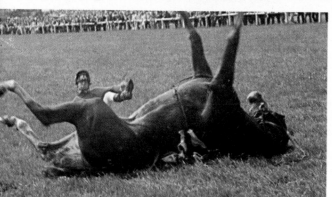

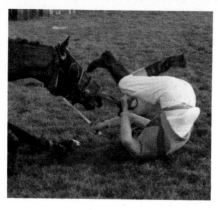

Above *After a fall such as this, the jockey is well within his rights to remount and continue the chase. In the case of a refusal, there are no fixed rules, the jockey can take the fence as many times as is worthwhile.*

Far left and left *Modern jockeys often use padding under their shirts to lessen the risks of injury.*

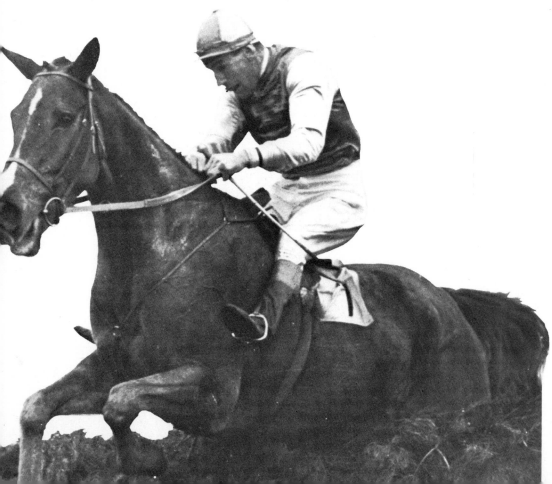

Left *Bryan Marshall riding Early Mist to success in the 1953 Grand National. The next year he was to prove just as successful on Royal Tan, to become one of a handful of jockeys to take the National in successive years. As with many retired jockeys, Marshall has set himself up as a trainer and has a steady stream of winners to his credit.*

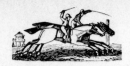

Tote starting-price of 444–1!

Seventeen horses took that fatal fence after Becher's Brook at the second or third attempt, to finish in one of the most sensational Grand Nationals of them all. Honey End, ridden by the champion jockey Josh Gifford, chased hard after Foinavon but could only make second place.

From flat racing to steeplechasing

One of the latest masters of Aintree's big fences and wide-open spaces is Red Rum. His racing career started with a dead-heat win in a race for two-year-olds run over 1006m (5 furlongs). He went on to win two more races on the flat over 1408m (7 furlongs). To date his record stands at over a score of races won, including two Grand Nationals and a Scottish National, and nearly £100,000 ($239,000) in prize money. And his career began with a lucky taxi ride.

Donald 'Ginger' McCain, Red Rum's trainer, had given up racing to set up a taxi and garage business. As the business prospered, he started to dabble in racing again, but purely on his own account. Having an eye for a good jumper, McCain bought horses that had broken down or which trainers did not want. Then, one day, McCain's taxi was booked by a self-made millionaire, Noel le Mare. On the drive along the Lancashire coast, the conversation turned to horses. By the end of the journey, Mr le Mare had commissioned McCain to buy him a horse for the Liverpool Grand National.

McCain bought Glenkiln at Doncaster Sales for £1000 ($2390) but when Noel le Mare heard the price he told McCain that the horse could not possibly be good enough. Searching for a better horse, McCain spotted Red Rum as he came second in the Scottish Grand National.

Red Rum changed to the le Mare colours for 6,000 guineas ($15,057) and Ginger McCain was faced with the job of preparing what was, by his standards, a very expensive horse for the Grand National. The training grounds were the sands at Southport.

At the same time, the now all-powerful Fred Winter stable, with a yard full of champions and potential world-beaters, was preparing a big Australian horse for the same race. A top-class horse in his own country and in England, Crisp was to challenge Red Rum at Aintree.

Brian Fletcher was chosen to ride Red Rum. Then 26-years-old, Fletcher had already won the National in 1968 when, in front of the packed Grandstands, he cruised across the line on 100–7 shot Red Alligator. His record in the race so far was five rides, one winner, one third, two falls and one refusal.

There are basically two types of jump-jockey. There is the pure race-rider, with a natural sense of balance, a mind that works like a whiplash and a will to win no matter what the cost to man or horse. Then there is the traditional horseman-jockey, who relies on his natural instinct as a horseman, his sympathy with the animal, his delicate hands and his ability to help the horse, should he run into trouble. Fletcher is the latter kind of jockey but also had the bravery and determination which Aintree demands.

Thirty-eight runners went to the starting post in ideal conditions, and the big Australian horse, Crisp, was the top weight. Red Rum was going at 9-to-1 with the featherweight of 65.77kg (10 stone 5lb). Fred Winter's charge Crisp set out to make nearly all the running and on the second circuit he was still leading, running at a tremendous speed.

Going for the second-last fence, Crisp was beginning to falter and Brian Fletcher and Red Rum made a spurt to catch Crisp. At the last fence, it looked as if Crisp might maintain his lead, although tired. But then, on landing, the agonizing run to the line was too much for Crisp. After galloping so intensely for so long, the big horse was now barely cantering. Brian Fletcher felt that Red Rum still had reserves of stamina and stormed him up the run-in to overhaul the almost-walking, worn-out figure of Crisp and flash past the post for Red Rum's first Grand National win.

In 1974, Red Rum returned to the scene of his triumph, still only a nine-year old. But this time, he had to carry a much heavier handicap—a top-weight of 76.20kg (12 stone), over the tough 7.24km (4½ miles). The Irish challenger L'Escargot was made favourite. On the second circuit, Red Rum skipped over Becher's Brook with Brian Fletcher safe in the saddle and went on to win with little difficulty. In 1975, however, L'Escargot prevented Red Rum creating a new record by beating him into second place.

International steeplechasing

Aintree is not the only place where steeplechasing laurels are fought for over fences by brave men and courageous horses. At Punchestown in Ireland the course has difficult fences, large banks and stone walls. The huge banks must be jumped with a very special technique, not too fast and not too slow, jump up on to the top, change legs for balance and jump off again.

Each country has its own supreme test of horse and rider. In Czechoslovakia, the Pardubice is the toughest jumping race in the racing calendar. Run more in the style of Dick Christian's days, it is a long, natural course with big fences, ditches, drop-fences and wide water-jumps which are very demanding for both horse and jockey. The Pardubice, with its thrills and spills, attracts riders from all over the world.

The Maryland Hunt Cup

At Glyndon in Maryland, the timber-jumping classic, The Maryland Hunt Cup, has been staged since 1894. A tough 6.43 km (5 mile) course over natural hunting-country, with post-and-rail or board-fences ranging from 1.14m (3ft 9in) to 1.47m (4ft 10in), with a water-jump spreading 1.83m (6ft) plus and a total of 22

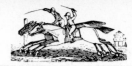

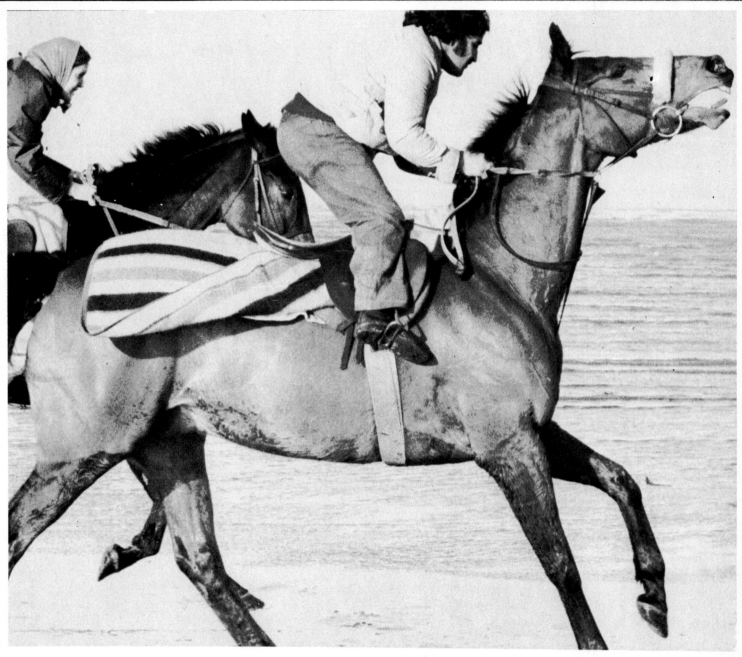

fences to be cleared before a winner is found. Superb 20th century steeplechase jockeys in the United States have made their names over this picturesque course. D Michael Smithwick has won it six times and Tommy Crompton Smith has taken the ribbons on no less than five occasions to date.

Grand Steeplechase de Paris

In France, the Parisian racegoers watch the sport of jumping at the Auteuil track, right in the middle of the city. What is known as a 'Park Course' in racing parlance, the sharp, twisty, fast track is full of surprises with a wide variety of fences.

In the Grand Steeplechase de Paris, horse and rider must cover 6·43km (4 miles) and negotiate 25 jumps laid out in a figure of eight. These include the Haie du Bull Finch, 0·76m (2ft 6in) of mud bank with 1·52m (5ft) of bullrushes on top. This the horses must jump through not over. And the Haie du Bank: a 0·76m (2ft 6in) hedge, six strides over a raised mound, descent over an 0·46m (18in) privet hedge with a 0·91m (3ft) drop. Then the Haie de la Grand Riviere: 5·49m (18ft) of water with a 0·76m (2ft 6in) hedge. This is followed by the Rail Ditch, 1·98m (6ft 6in) of gaping open ditch followed by a brush fence of 1·68m (5ft 6in). Then the Haie de l'Oxer, described as two small brush fences with an 2·44m (8ft) spread but looking threatening to horse and jockey.

It was on this course that Fred Winter held the French 'Turfistes' spell-bound by his powers of horsemanship. He was riding the very successful English steeplechaser, Mandarin, in the Grand Steeple.

From jockey to trainer

The success story of Fred Winter is legendary. The son of one of Britain's leading trainers, he

Above *Profile of one of the latest and most consistent heroes of Aintree, Red Rum, out training on the sands of Southport with stable companion Crocodilla.*

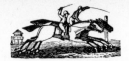

One of the most successful
National Hunt jockeys to
make the transition to
training, Fred Winter.
Below *Taking Kilmore
over the last fence of the
1962 Grand National to win
by 10 lengths.* **Far right**
*Riding Saffron Tartan in
the 1961 Cheltenham
Gold Cup.*

Right *The legendary Arkle,
in 35 outings he was only
unplaced once.*

Bottom *The beautiful
Cotswold setting for the
Cheltenham Gold Cup.*

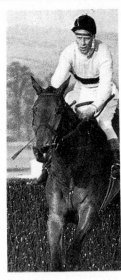

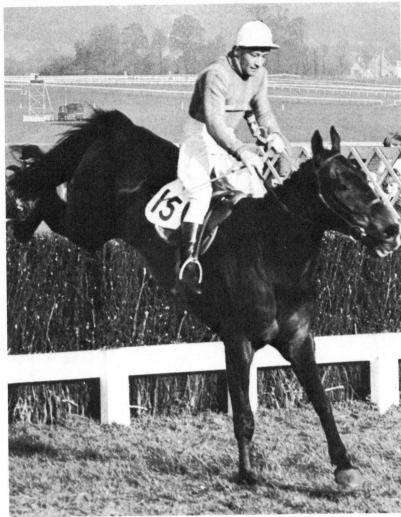

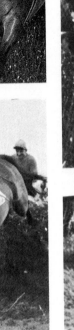

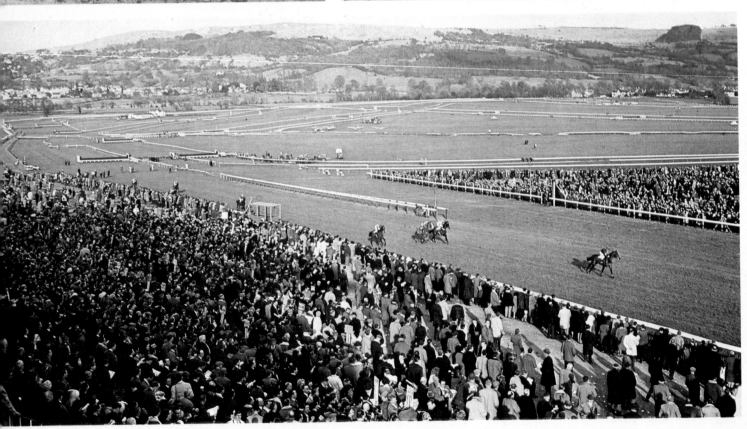

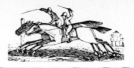

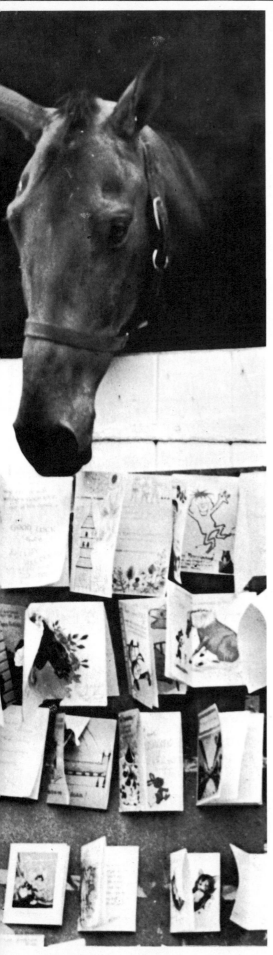

rode in almost 4500 races over 17 seasons, for ten of which he was Champion Jockey. Of his almost 1000 winning rides, the Grand National accounts for two, with two Cheltenham Gold Cups and one Grand Steeplechase de Paris.

His winning of the Grand Steeplechase de Paris was one of his great, successful, brilliant and hair-raising feats of riding. The head-strong Mandarin, winner of the Cheltenham Gold Cup, broke his bit at the fourth fence and Fred had to ride the remaining 21 fences of the twisty sharp track with no bridle. With no visible means of support but some help from his friend and fellow jockey, Monsieur Daumas, whose 'boxing in' of the bridleless Mandarin enabled Fred to follow the complicated race-strip, Mandarin won in front of 50,000 cheering French people.

The legendary Arkle

On the 'Park-tracks' of Cheltenham, the Ascot of the steeplechasing scene, and the fashionable London tracks, Arkle and Pat Taaffe, two more 'greats' of steeplechasing, captured the public imagination. Arkle one of the most popular steeplechasers of all time never ran in the Grand National. His owner, Anne, Duchess of Westminster, thought the chances of her horse getting injured were too great. In the old days the Grand National prize was the only one worth winning but in post-war years there were plenty of large prizes for the talented fencer, such as the Cheltenham Gold Cup and the King George VI Chase, so that it is not necessary to enter the National.

Arkle became an equine super-star. He could draw crowds to racecourses that were every Clerk of the Course's dream. His fans would gather at the starting-gate to get a closer look at him. He had that special charisma and he knew it. As if playing to his public, he would put in his biggest and most dramatic leap at the fence in front of the stands and then cock his ears and look for the next one. Arkle was one of the only jumpers who were applauded by racegoers each time he jumped a fence or appeared in the paddock.

Arkle won the Cheltenham Gold Cup three times and the King George VI Chase once. The thrilling battles between the small, tough Arkle and the big, long-striding Mill House were a top-of-the-bill feature of Cheltenham and the major tracks of England and Ireland. Trained in Ireland by the great Tom Dreaper, the giant-killing gelding was ridden throughout his career by one of the finest jump-jockeys Ireland has produced, Pat Taaffe.

Arkle's end was a tragic one. While attempting to win the King George VI Chase for the second time in December 1966, this normally agile jumper hit a guard-rail going into a fence and cracked his pedal bone and could never race again.

Thousands of letters and telegrams arrived at Tom Dreaper's stables from all over the world. Television-crews and journalists queued to inter-

Below *Arkle is probably the most famous steeplechaser never to have run in the Grand National. His owner, the Duchess of Westminster preferred not to risk her great horse over Aintree's fences.*

Left *However, the normally agile jumper broke a bone in his foot at Kempton Park on Boxing Day 1966 and never raced again. Get well cards poured in from all over the world.*

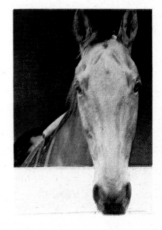

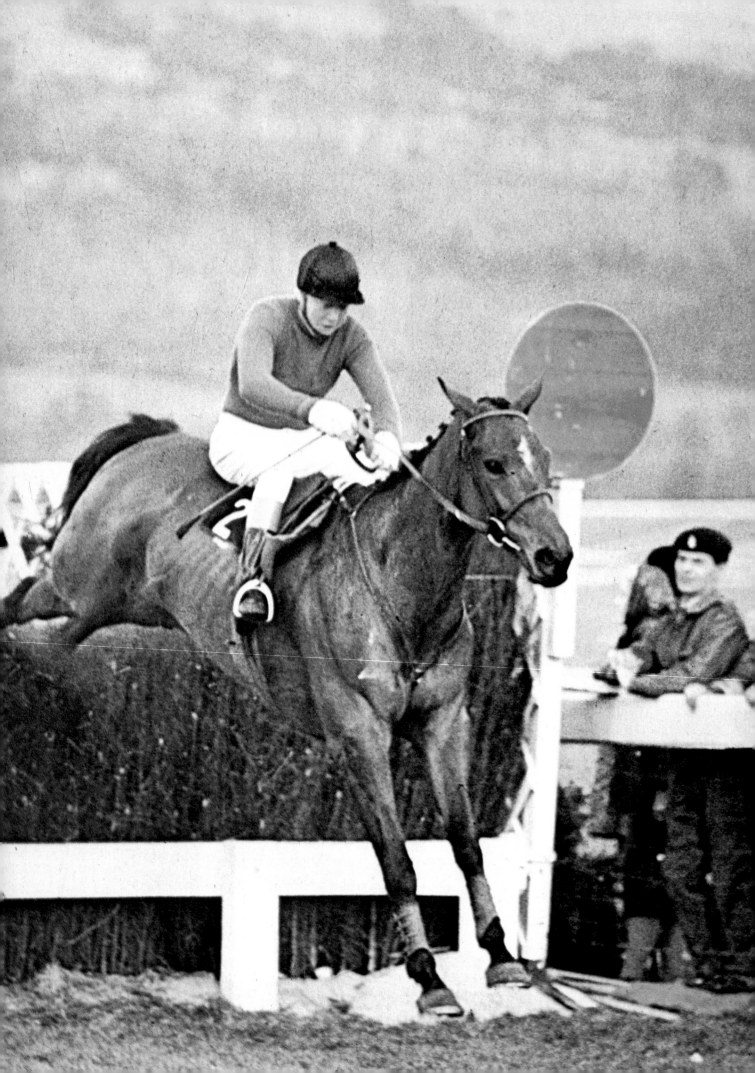

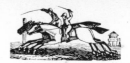

view the greatest park-chaser of all time. Arkle had won 27 races worth £73,617 ($176,680) and had become a national hero.

A nursery for steeplechasers

Most steeplechasers start their careers in Hurdle-racing. These use smaller and flimsier obstacles, jumped at near flat-racing speed. They take the form of a sheep-hurdle with gorse or spruce interwoven in the wooden cross-bars, and the top-rail is covered with rubber. They are staked into the turf and set at an angle away from the horses. In some countries, they take the form of small brush-fences or plank-fences, but the principle is the same: to encourage fast, slick jumping.

Not all hurdle-racers are destined for the bigger jumps. Many, particularly ex-flat racehorses, specialize in this exciting form of racing. Hurdle-

Opposite *One of the most popular jockeys both with the crowds and with his fellow jockeys, Terry Biddlecombe, rides Woodland Venture to victory in the 1967 Cheltenham Gold Cup.*

Below and below left *Three times champion National Hunt jockey, Stan Mellor, takes Gay Bruce over in a 1970 handicap hurdles. Hurdling forms a perfect training ground for steeplechasers and many ex-flat racing horses specialize in this form of jumping.*

Bottom *Some great finishes at Cheltenham.* **Left** *Cottage Rake takes the lead from Happy Home.* **Centre** *Pas Seul and Lochroe in 1960.* **Right** *The great rivals, Arkle and Mill House in 1965.*

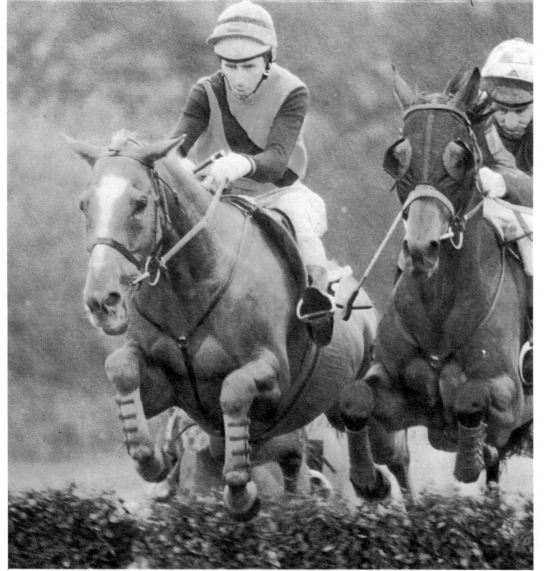

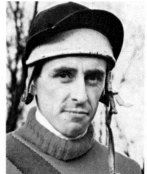

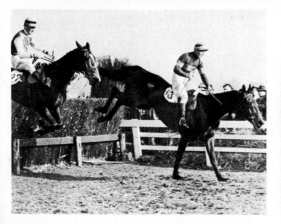

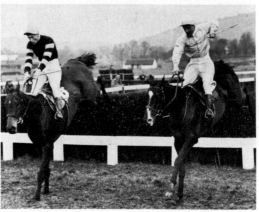

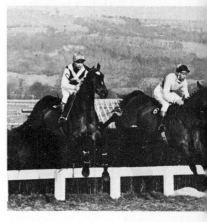

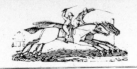

racing has produced its own special stars, such as Sir Ken and Cottage Rake, winners of the Cheltenham Champion Hurdle several times, Salmon Spray, another Champion title-winner, the consistent National Spirit, one of the record-holders for the number of hurdle-races won. It has its own artists in the saddle too, like George Duller, Harry Sprague, Geordie Ramshaw and Jimmy Uttley.

Persian War

In recent years, hurdle-racing in England was dominated by the long-striding Persian War. A strong, good-looking dark bay gelding, Persian War was first brought out as a crack three-year old hurdler by trainer Tom Masson, and ridden by Bunny Hicks. He was then purchased by Mr Henry Alper and sent to the Epsom ex-flat-race jockey, Brian Swift to be trained. It was here that he struck up a special relationship with crack hurdle-rider, Jimmy Uttley. Jimmy was to be his jockey throughout his glorious career.

It was during his years at Epsom with Brian Swift that Persian War really dominated hurdle-racing. Not an easy horse to train, Brian Swift produced him, perfectly tuned, to win several important and valuable hurdle-races, and to take the coveted Champion Hurdle at Cheltenham on no less than three occasions. He was voted race-horse of the year, books were written about him and even a film was made of him.

Twentieth century developments

The face of horse jumping is changing, with a new-style fencing jockey and steeplechaser coming on to the scene. In American, French and English steeplechasing and hurdling, the influence of the flat-race jockey is having a great effect on techniques and standards. Very few of the jockeys come from the amateur ranks or the hunting-field. Most are now ex-flat jockeys who have become too heavy and turn to jumping with considerable success. Some are flat-race riders who like to mix hurdle-racing with flat-racing. These jockeys are more professional than some of the hurdle and steeplechase riders of the past.

A new-style horse has also come into the game. With rising costs and increasing prize-money through sponsorship, owners are now keeping their horses in training for longer periods. Some owners race them both on the flat and over hurdles, while some others send them on from hurdling to steeplechasing with increasing success. This all-rounder type of horse, which often goes on to become a successful steeplechaser, is more akin to a flat-racer than to the generally accepted jumper of the past. In the old days, when the jumping-game was more of an amateur sport than the specialized, professional sport it is today, the steeplechaser was of a traditional type. It was usually a half-bred (a thoroughbred stallion crossed with a non-thoroughbred mare) or a near thoroughbred that was not registered in the General Stud Book. He was usually a big, long-striding horse with a lot of 'bone' and generally more heavy-framed than his flat-racing counterpart. This was the type that the steeplechase owner or trainer would look for but as a breed it was non-existent. As jump-racing became more popular, a type of thoroughbred evolved that was genetically a pure-bred but with characteristics that set him apart from the flat-racer type. This

Opposite page *Josh Gifford riding Aursibio in the 1970 KP Hurdle at Kempton Park.*

Below right *The new style jockey, greatly influenced by flat racing techniques, now rides with much shorter stirrups than his counterpart of a hundred years ago and distributes his weight so as to interfere to the minimum in the horse's natural racing action.*

Below *The moment they've all been striving for – trainer Fred Rimell leads the victorious Gay Trip in to the winner's enclosure.*

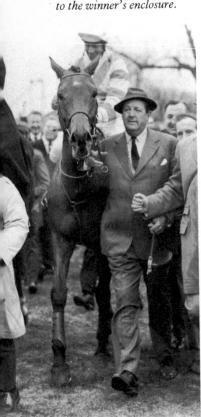

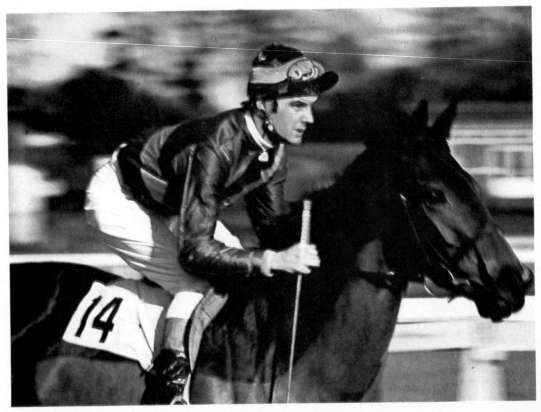

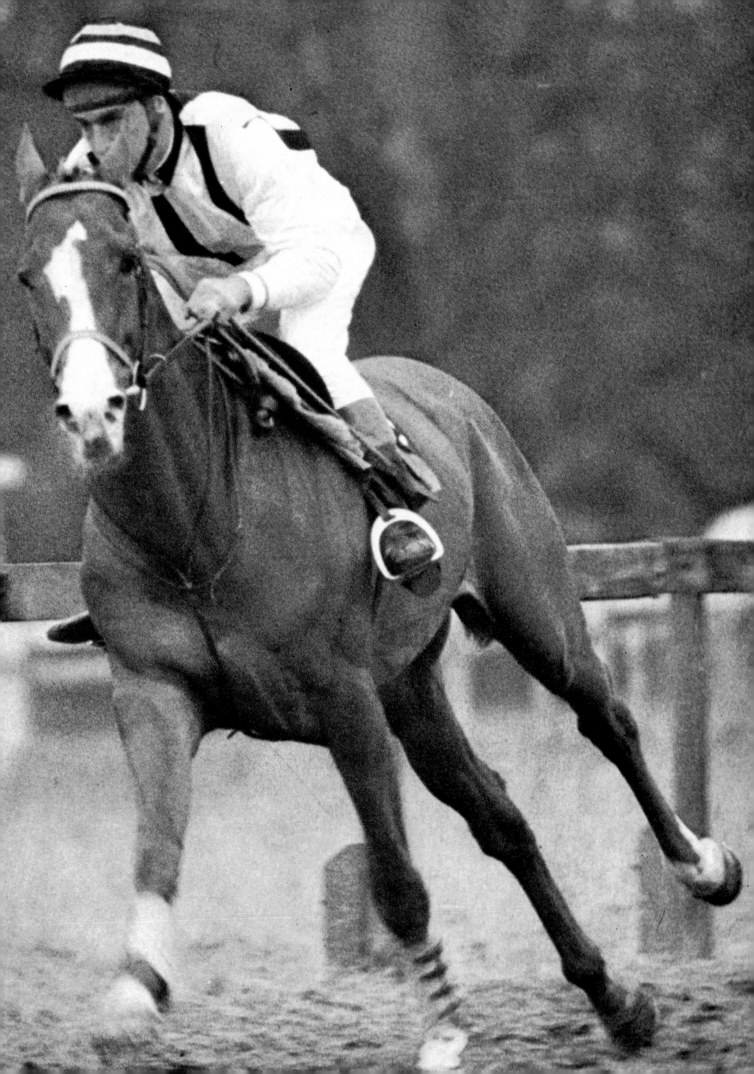

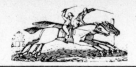

has become a sort of sub-breed under the title of Anglo-Irish Steeplechaser.

One of the best examples of the Anglo-Irish steeplechaser was the great Arkle, a horse specifically bred for the jumping-game. Indeed, his sire, Archive, although a classically bred horse, with a poor racing record, established himself as a leading sire of jumpers. Arkle was not a handsome horse in the technical sense and yet his conformation was perfect for the tough game of steeplechasing. His body was strong, powerful and active; his chest was broad and deep; his legs were short but well boned and, the most important asset for a jumper, his forearm and second thigh carried plenty of muscle. Add to this his natural competitive spirit and Arkle is the prototype for the steeplechasing type. Not all jumpers, of course, can or do resemble Arkle. Many very good steeplechasers are nearer in looks and bloodline to the flat-racer.

Steeplechasing and hurdle-racing at a very high standard is unique to England and Ireland. Here, it is no longer the 'country cousin' of flat-racing but an equal partner in the spectator-sport industry of racing. Nowhere else in the world is the sport so professional and concentrated as it is in the British Isles. In France, where short tracks and uniform fences are used, it is mainly a 'gap-filler' on the race-card and a sport for the failed flat-racer. In America, the fences are low and made of 'brush', or the amateur version, which is run over timber fences in Hunt events, predominates. In other parts of the world, such as Australia and New Zealand, attempts have been made to introduce steeplechasing but it never really gathered momentum. Apart from a small band of keen semi-amateurs, the sport is almost non-existent outside the United Kingdom.

There has always been a small percentage of blue-blooded horses in hurdle-racing, but in recent seasons, we have seen more of the better-bred horses taking the valuable Handicap and Cup steeplechases on the park-courses such as Cheltenham, Sandown, Auteuil and Belmont in the United States. But as yet they have not had much success in the more demanding 'natural' races such as the Grand National 24-year period from 1946 to 1969. For example, seven winners of the Grand National were half-breds. During the same period, all the winners of the Cheltenham Gold Cup were pure aristocratic thoroughbreds.

The modern horse and the modern rider have come to stay, and the game is prospering with each season. The new-style fencing jockey rides with a shorter leather. Like his flat-race counterpart, he sits closer and tighter to his horse as they zip along the race-strip over fences which are more uniform but just as stiff as ever.

From Hong Kong to New York, race-fans flock to see the jumping game, and although winning may be the aim, the element of danger keeps the fraternity cemented together in the spirit of sportsmanship.

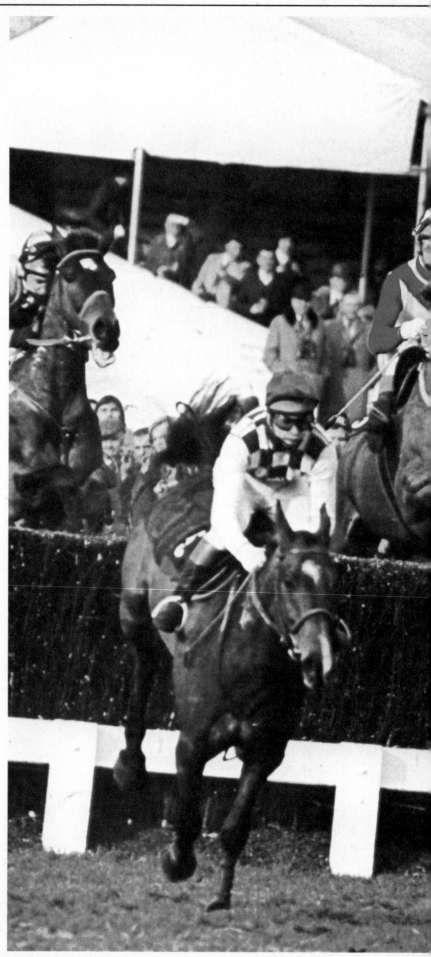

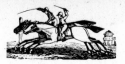

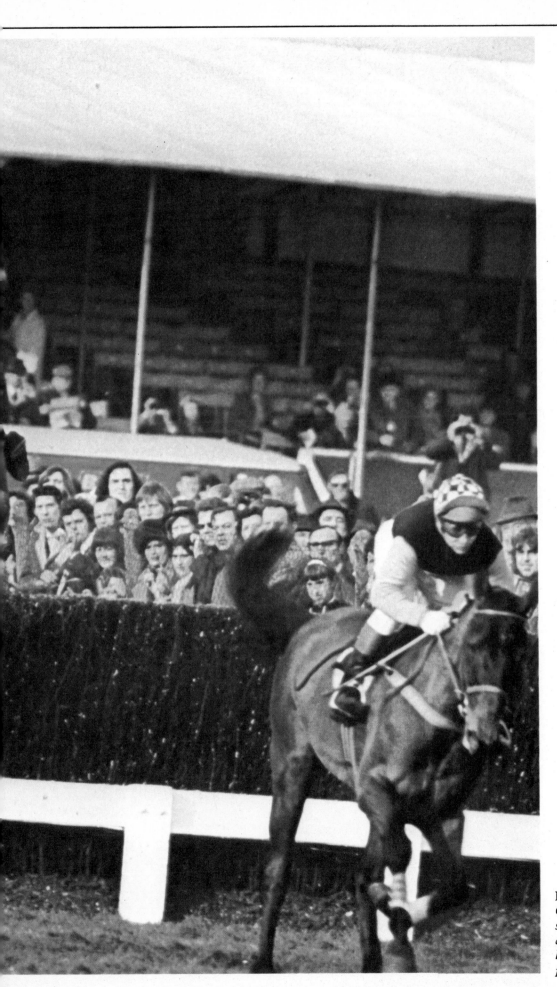

Left *The 1974 Cheltenham Gold Cup. Taking the second fence The Dikler and Captain Christy. In the lead High Ken hotly pursued by Pendil.*

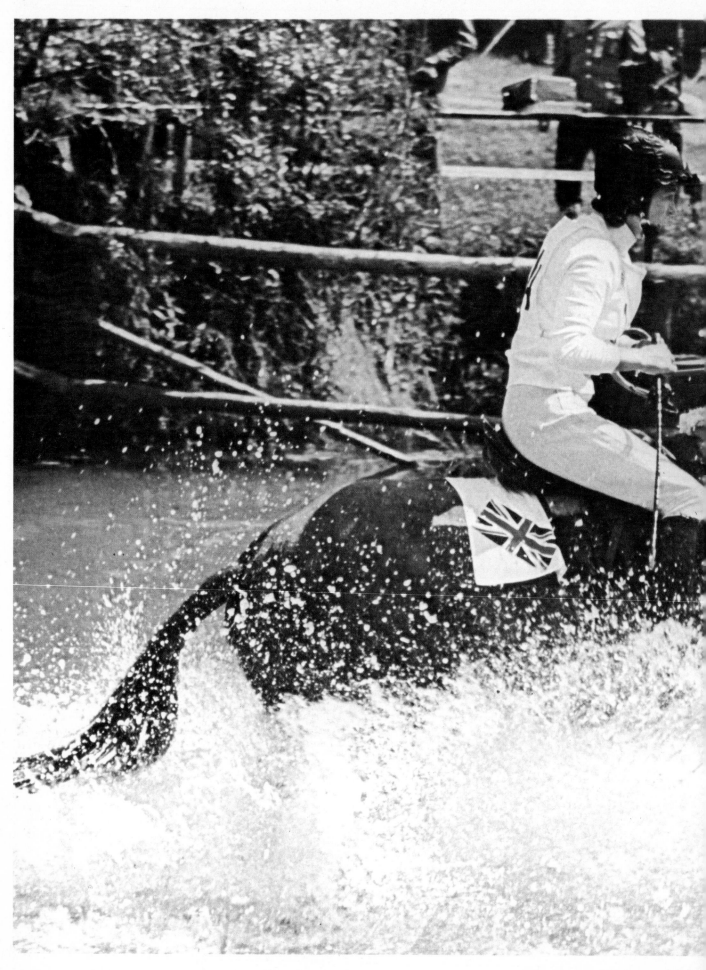

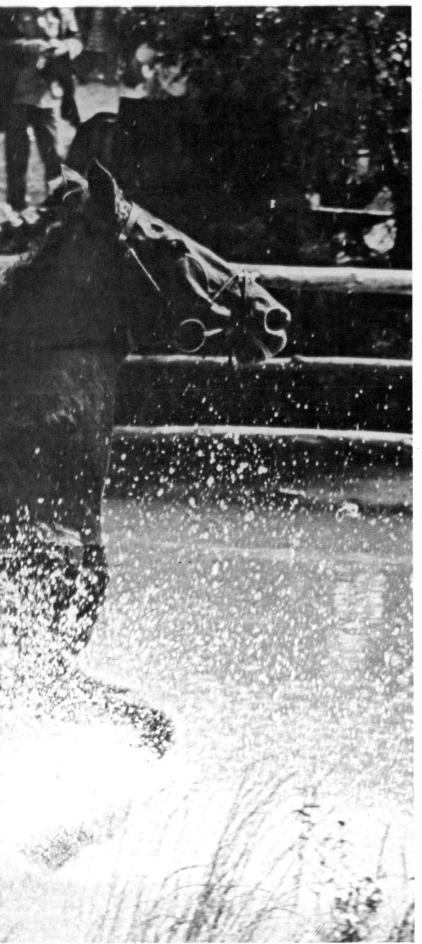

The Three Day Event

Combined training, also known as three-day eventing and horse-trialing, comes from the era of the great military riding academies. The famous schools of Saumur and Fontainebleau in France, Pinerolo in Italy, Madrid, Spain, West Point in the United States and Weedon, England were the closed chapels of advanced equitation up to the early part of this century.

The Military Academies

While the part of the civilian population interested in horses was still riding across country hunting fox or deer, galloping around racecourses, or jumping their mounts over coloured poles on the village green, the young officer was being drilled in the arts of equitation according to the narrow doctrines of an army manual. The combined training system was part-and-parcel of military equestrianism and each academy had its own style, and its own interpretation of the ultimate test of horse and rider.

What was this system? Basically, the idea was to create situations to test the officer and his charger in varying conditions and in all aspects of riding. An experienced officer would train his charger himself, so the system tested not only his ability as a horseman but also his talent as a trainer. Due in large part to these military schools, jumping and galloping to order became a sport—a sport that each year is becoming more popular and more international.

Marathon of equestrian sports

Combined training displays equitations's finest skills. It is the field of competition which demands that horse and rider demonstrate all their combined talents, and all the disciplines which the art represents. This is the marathon of equestrian sports. The three-day event combination of horse and rider must be able to rely on their reserves of courage, their flexibility of mind and the reflexes of their trained bodies. Months of training are required before they reach the standard set in the field of competition. And then horse and rider never know when they will rendezvous with success or failure. Trainer and rider, often the same person, must live with the horse, understand his nature and have total confidence in his ability. Their dependence on each other is complete, their unity and cohesion are

The most spectacular jump on the course and the one that attracts the largest crowd – the water jump.

Right *Although one of the toughest of equestrian sports, the three-day event allows women to compete on equal terms with the men and they do outstandingly well. Here, Sheila Willcox on High and Mighty on whom she won the Badminton Horse Trials in 1957 and 1958.*

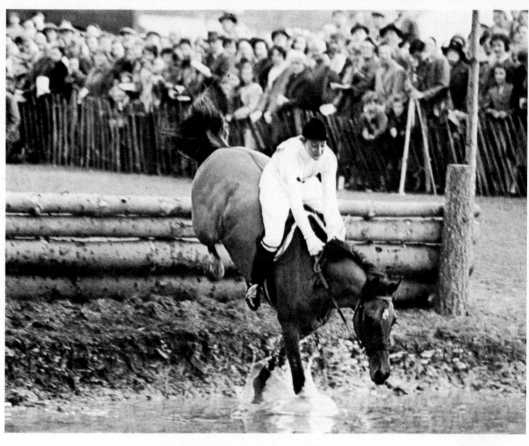

vital to their common purpose. These are the truths of combined training and the reasons why this sport is the most demanding, the most testing and possibly the most satisfying for the true horse enthusiast.

In its early days, three-day eventing was a minority pastime. But since World War II it has enriched the equestrian scene and become an enjoyable and widespread national, and international, sport. Known under its various titles according to country, it is perhaps the French term Concours Complet d'Equitation which describes it the most accurately, although it is also known generally on the Continent as the Militaire, which pays due respect to its origins.

The three phases

The combined-training competition is basically divided into three phases. First, an obedience test, the dressage phase. Then, a speed and endurance test: the roads-and-tracks, steeplechase and cross-country phase. And finally, a test of soundness and ability to continue after the tough cross-country section: the show-jumping phase over smallish, coloured fences within the confines of an arena. Between each phase the horses are subjected to a stiff veterinary examination to prevent a courageous and willing horse being asked to do too much. The event takes place over three days in senior competition only and is scaled down to take one or two days in the novice and intermediate grades. Badminton, Burghley and Fontainebleau are the three main venues for the Senior European competitions.

Day One

The first day of a senior three-day event begins with the dressage test. This is performed in a rectangular arena with lettered marker-boards showing the precise points at which turns and other movements must be executed. For example, the long centre-line is always marked at one end by 'C' and at the other by 'A', and the short centre-line by the letters 'E' and 'B' at either end, and so on round the arena. The dressage test is not a difficult one by international dressage standards, but it is designed to test the horse's obedience and readiness to go forward willingly, and the rider's knowledge, control and expertise in the use of the aids (the system of signals used to control the horse based on the rider's hands, seat and legs). The panel is looking not only for accuracy in carrying out movements but also for grace and fluency. The panel marks are given in minus quantities, directly related to accepted international co-efficients. In the early days of eventing few competitors achieved very high markings in a dressage test, or if one did, it gave him a commanding lead going into the other phases. Nowadays, the standard of competition is such that only a mere handful of points will separate the leaders at the end of the first day and will not affect the final markings to the great extent it once did.

Day Two

The second day is the speed and endurance test. This starts off with a laid-out trail of roads and tracks over about 6½km (approx. 4 miles). The

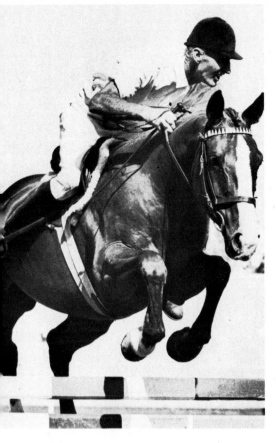

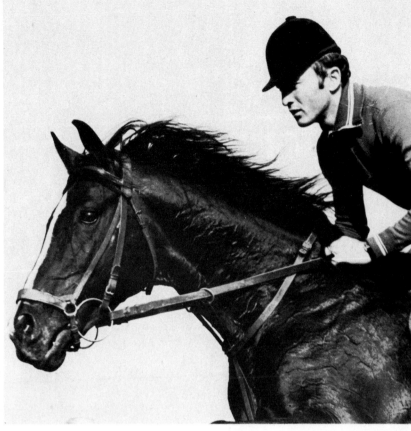

pace is set at 240m per minute (9 miles per hour), a speed which is not all that easy for a horse to maintain consistently. This stage is usually done at the trot. A minimum time is allowed, which on average works out at around 25 minutes. Penalties are given at the rate of one point for each minute or fraction of a minute outside the time allowed. If a competitor is five or more minutes over the set time, he is eliminated. No bonus points are given for completing the first roads-and-tracks phase in a fast time, but this does give the competitor an advantage as he goes into the next phase, the steeplechase.

The steeplechase course is usually around 4km (2½ miles), with at least 12 racing type fences. The time allowed is six minutes, which gives an average pace of 600m per minute (22 miles per hour). Bonus points are given at the rate of 0·8 point per second, and penalties are calculated on the same basis. The bonus points are subtracted from the dressage score and any penalties gained on the first roads-and-tracks. Penalty points are added to these two other scores.

By the time the steeplechase phase is reached there are already some clear leaders. This is where the ability and experience of the rider are at a premium. He must now be capable of estimating his horse's potential, using it fully but at the same time avoiding putting too much strain on him, as there are still three more very gruelling phases to be completed. The first of these last three is only found in top-class international competitions, and is a second roads-and-tracks or endurance test. But this one is normally much

longer than the first, some 12·8km (8 miles) to be covered at the trot and within 50 minutes. But this time there are no bonus points for going quickly, only the advantage of giving the horse more time to get his second wind.

The next phase of the three-day event is the cross-country section. This is the most spectacular part of the sport, and for those taking part, the real 'meat' of the competition. At this stage the pressure is really exerted on the rider and his mount. Any weaknesses in the horse's training schedule will show up. The rider's ability and courage will be scrupulously tested.

Before starting the test, the rider will have walked the course to study all the obstacles. He will look at them from all angles and check the state of the ground going into the fence and on the landing side. He will study the height and width and the distance from one fence to another. He will decide where to go fast and where to slow down. He will work out his track, his approaches and try to imagine in his own mind how the course is going to 'ride' and where he may have difficulties.

The horses must be passed by a veterinary surgeon before they can start the cross-country run. Each is tested for soundness of limb and heart; they are inspected for injuries and any signs of over-fatigue. Only when the veterinary surgeons are fully satisfied that the horse is fit and well and able to carry on, will the rider be allowed to depart for the toughest phase of all, the cross-country.

The cross-country course is usually some 8km

Above *In the USSR equestrianism is growing in popularity. In contrast to the practice in the West, the USSR provides training facilities for their riders at a very early age. Here Ferdinand Kibizov, Master of Sports at the republican equestrian school in Ordzhonikidze, takes a jump.*

Above left *Australian Bill Roycroft. Not only was he a member of two medal winning Olympic teams and the first Australian to win the Badminton Three Day Trials, in 1965 he finished third to the great Arkle and Mill House in the Cheltenham Gold Cup steeplechase on his own horse, Stoney Crossing.*

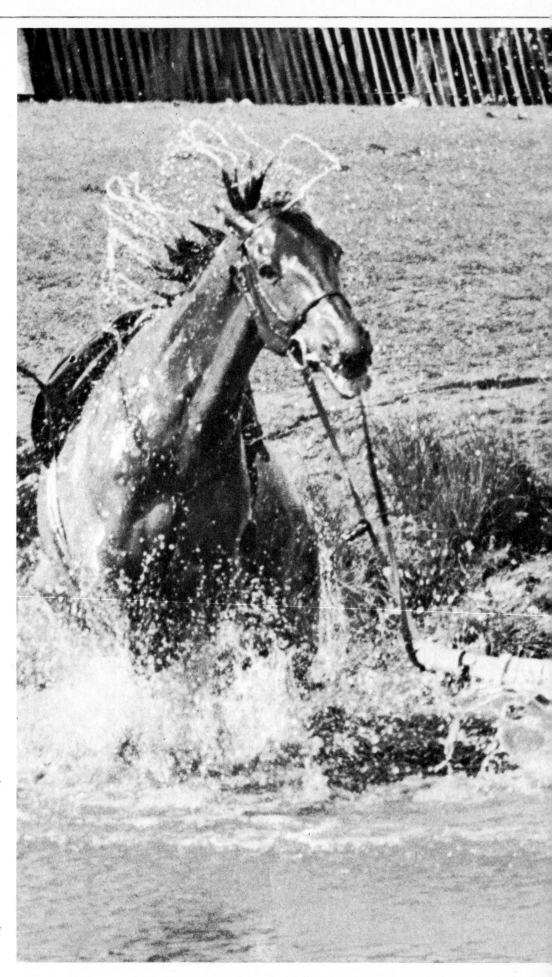

Right *Water jumps pose some of the greatest problems to horse and rider. Here Farewell has an uncertain landing and unseats his rider Mrs M F Jones.*

Far right *Some of the most outstanding riders in this sport come from Australia. Laurie Morgan, the Australian captain takes a fence to win at Badminton in 1961 on Salad Days.*

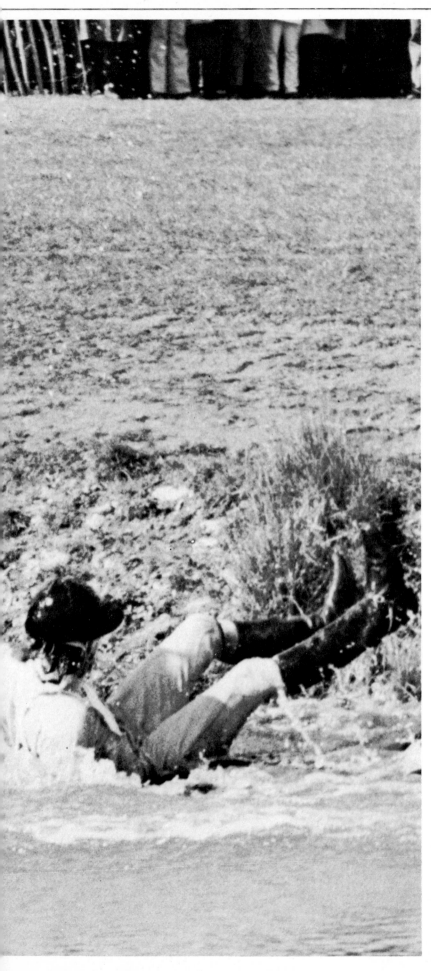

(5 miles) in length, with between 30 and 35 obstacles. These are fixed, solid fences, varying in height around 0·9–1·2m (3–4ft); the width of some fences can be as much as 3·0–3·4m (10–11ft). Water-jumps (fences followed by water such as a stream as opposed to a fence followed by a lake), stretch some 3·7–4·3m (12–14ft). Combinations can be doubles (two fences) or trebles (three fences) made up of bars or oxers, and these can have spreads of over 1·8m (6ft). All these must be covered at a speed exceeding 400m per minute (15 miles per hour). The total time for the cross-country stage is 16 minutes.

The competitor is awarded bonus points for time gained, at the rate of 0·4 point for one second. If, for example, a competitor covered an international track in 12 minutes 37 seconds, he would be awarded 81·2 points. These are bonus points and are therefore subtracted from penalty points. So a horse and rider who have collected heavy penalties in the dressage but go well and fast across country, can offset their poor standard of dressage. In top-class eventing, the key to success is to be above-average in the dressage, thus going into the other phases with as few penalties as possible, and to be as close to brilliant as possible in the cross-country. In this way, if a particular horse and rider are in the lead or near the top markings by the end of the second day, even a moderate last-day performance could be good enough to win the competition.

Penalties can be collected on the cross-country phase and they are calculated on a time factor. For completing the course over the maximum 32 minutes allowed, elimination usually follows. For a refusal at a fence the penalty points are as follows: first refusal 20 penalties, second refusal 40 penalties and for a third at the same obstacle,

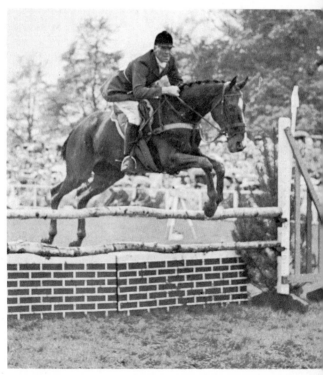

elimination. The fall of horse or rider costs 60 points (a third fall on the cross-country bringing elimination). Four penalties are given if a horse or rider displaces the red and white markers showing which way, or where, an obstacle is to be jumped. The same penalties are picked up if the horse or rider hits the barriers or rails marking the track and approaches to fences. If a rider takes the wrong course or jumps out of sequence, he is eliminated. But if he goes back and corrects his mistake, he can carry on but, of course, picks up time penalties. Equally, if a contestant jumps a fence twice, then elimination is once again the price he pays.

The fascination of the cross-country phase in eventing is not so much the massive dimensions of the fences as the variety of the obstacles and the approaches to them. At the 1974 World Championship, held at Burghley House near Stamford, England, one of the features of the course was a fence called the Trout Hatchery. This was a steep-sided bank leading down to a natural post-and-rails in front of a small lake. There was a long approach which meant that the horses were going quite fast, looking for time-bonuses and, although the fence itself was not very big, a number of competitors found that errors of judgement not only involved a loss of points but also, in many cases, a gratuitous bathing in the lake.

As with each fence throughout the course, the competitor was faced with several problems or 'questions' as they are called in the sport. He could slow to a trot, come down the little bank, 'pop' over the rails into the water and then gallop on again. Or he could decide to do the opposite and come at it fast and ask his mount to take off at the top of the slope, stretch out over the rails and land well out into the water, gaining precious time.

This decision will probably already have been made when the rider walked the course beforehand. Remember, he has probably already covered something like 64km (about 40 miles) on his own two feet studying the course, working out the approaches, listening to the advice of others or, if he is a member of a team, arguing and discussing all its peculiarities with the captain of the team. He has worked for this day for months, even years, and the decisions he makes the night before will either bring grief or success.

But on the actual day previous plans may have to be hastily revised, exerting even more pressure on a rider. He waits for his turn, trying to think of other things so as to remain in a calm, collected frame of mind. The first riders have already started and as they finish, they relate their experiences. In the collecting-ring, friends tell of what has happened to other competitors. Tension builds up as well-laid plans have to be revised quickly and decisively.

Then the competitor's name is called and horse and rider set out into the countryside to face 30 difficult fences. The panorama the horseman

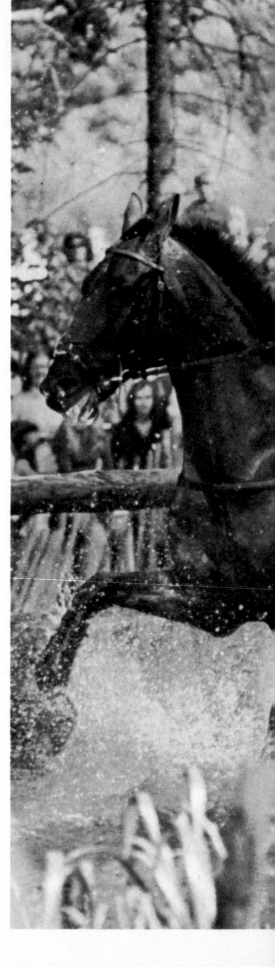

The 1974 World Champion, Bruce Davidson takes Irish Cap through the water jump at Burghley on the way to taking his title.

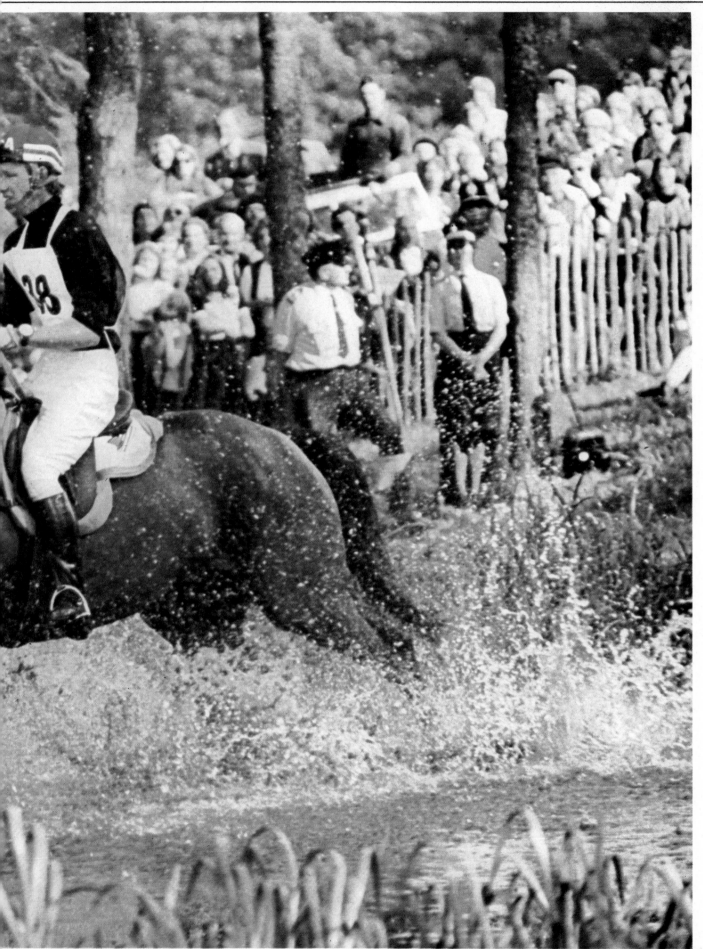

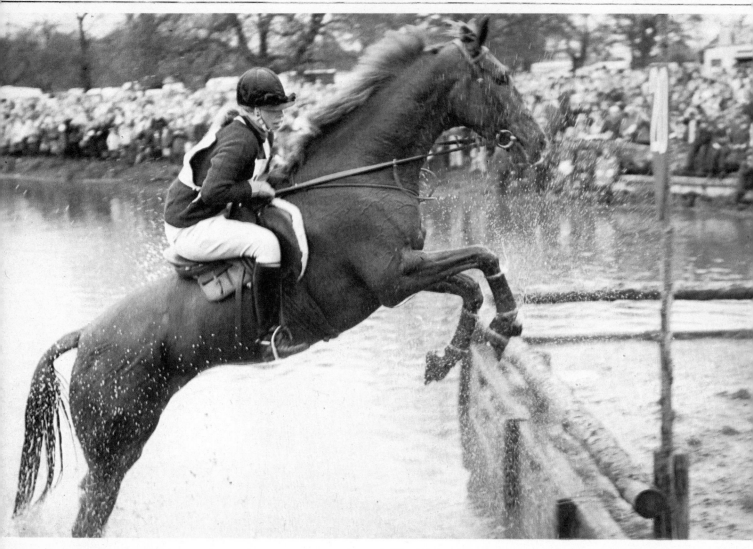

scans between the ears of his galloping mount can be a daunting one. Valleys come and go, woods and ploughed land, open fields, with fences situated everywhere. On top of hills, in ditches, lakes, across roads, into sheep-pens on awkward turns, narrow slides down to solid fences set on the banks of streams or rivers. These are the test of long hours of training. Questions race through the rider's mind, 'Has the horse enough scope for the really big fence on the course?'; 'Is my speed right?'; 'Has he got the stamina to keep this up after all those roads and tracks, and the steeple-chase?' Then, almost suddenly, the open stretch of the run-in appears. The concentration, fear, daring, are an inevitable but exhilarating feature of the cross-country test.

Day Three

The final day is taken up with the show-jumping phase. In the old days of eventing, when the sport was the preserve of the military, this phase had nothing to do with show-jumping as it is now practised. It was just a small course of natural obstacles and the object was to prove that horse and rider could still complete a simple obedience test after two such gruelling days. In other words, although pushed to the maximum, they could

still call upon reserves of stamina if required.

In modern competitions, the third day is much nearer a conventional show-jumping contest. The fences are coloured and laid out in an arena, but the rules are not exactly the same as in show-jumping. Five penalties are incurred for knocking a fence down and 15 for a fall of horse or rider. Once again, three refusals at the same obstacle mean elimination. The required speed is 350m per minute (13 miles per hour) and the track is usually 732m (2402ft) long. The fences are relatively low, being of novice show-jumping standard, but the course builder purposely creates a course involving numerous changes of direction, to test the horse's obedience as well as his ability to jump coloured fences.

The growth of modern eventing

Three-day eventing has been one of the three equestrian events in the Olympic Games since it was first added to the modern programme in 1912. This has been a popular sport on the Continent for many years but when Great Britain entered a team in the 1936 Games, the event did not even exist in England.

It was not until the 1948 Olympic Games at Wembley, England (the three-day event was held mainly at the Army centre, Aldershot) that the sport really started to gain popularity. The two surviving English riders finished very high in the final classification and as the sport was being seen in this country for the first time, amateurs of horse competition took to it instantly. Britain and Ireland, with their long tradition of hunting across natural country, had a ready-made stock of horses and riders whose aptitude and ability were almost tailor-made for the sport of combined training.

The Duke of Beaufort, a keen equestrian and Master of Foxhounds, was very impressed by the possibilities of three-day eventing as a sport and a spectacle. So in the spring of 1949, he created the Badminton Horse Trials in the magnificent park of his ancestral home, Badminton House, Gloucestershire, marking a date in the sporting calendar that was to become as important to the international horse trials scene as the Grand National is to racing men.

The cross-country course at Badminton is one of the most formidable on the world eventing circuit. It is a fast course and tends to favour the 'blood' (thoroughbred or near-thoroughbred)

horse and the skilful, classical rider. In that first year the winner was Capt J Shedden riding Golden Willow, but since then the competition has become very popular with the international stars of the sport. Many have come to conquer Badminton, only to be conquered by it.

Sheila Willcox

Gradually more and more civilians took up the sport and, because it offered no material rewards, the 'amateur' atmosphere has remained to this day. The first real English star of three-day eventing was the talented and determined Sheila Willcox, a self-taught, blonde-haired horsewoman who when she turned her attention to horse trials, purchased a seven-year-old Irish gelding to enter the Badminton Trials. This was not only an unusually-bred horse, but an unusually-coloured one. It was a dun gelding with a dark stripe and donkey-lines on his legs, and half-Arab, half-Highland blood running through his veins. He was called Chips at home, and High and Mighty on the field of competition. Horse and rider were to become equestrian legends in their own lifetimes and caused a revolution in the sport.

Below *Clearing the fence with style. Most of the fences on the second day's cross-country test are solid and designed to try every facet of the horse's abilities.*

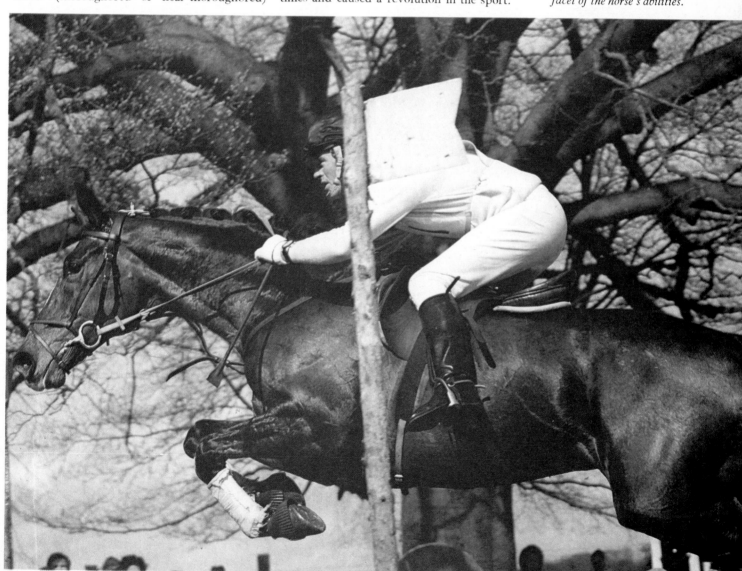

Right *The young Sheila Willcox on her Irish bred High and Mighty. It was largely due to her success on this horse that women were accepted into this exacting sport.*

Below *Lucinda Prior-Palmer takes Be Fair perfectly over a fence to win the 1973 Badminton Horse Trials. The obstacles in the third day's trials are designed for the sole purpose of testing the horse's suppleness and obedience after the exertions of the previous day's cross country event.*

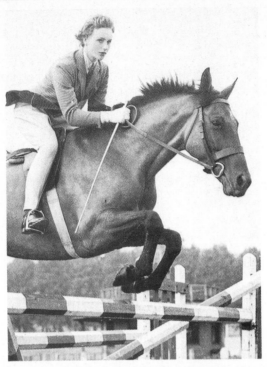

They first burst on to the international scene in 1956 in Turin, where they were members of the winning British team and took the individual winners' ribbons. In that same year, Sheila had also finished second at Badminton to Lieutenant-Colonel Frank Weldon. To come second to Frank Weldon and his great horse Kilbarry after so little experience was no mean achievement. Kilbarry was an Irish-bred gelding who did full-time duty with the King's Troop of the Royal Horse Artillery. Besides winning Badminton twice, and going to the Olympic Games at Stockholm in 1956 with the Gold-medal-winning British team, he was also the first British horse to win an individual Bronze medal, with Frank Weldon riding him. This great horse regrettably came to a tragic end, breaking his neck at a one-day event.

In 1957 Sheila Willcox and High and Mighty took the winning honours at Badminton, repeating their victory the following year. Then in 1959 she rode the winner for the third consecutive time, a record which has yet to be beaten. This time Sheila was now Mrs Waddington and her mount was Airs and Graces.

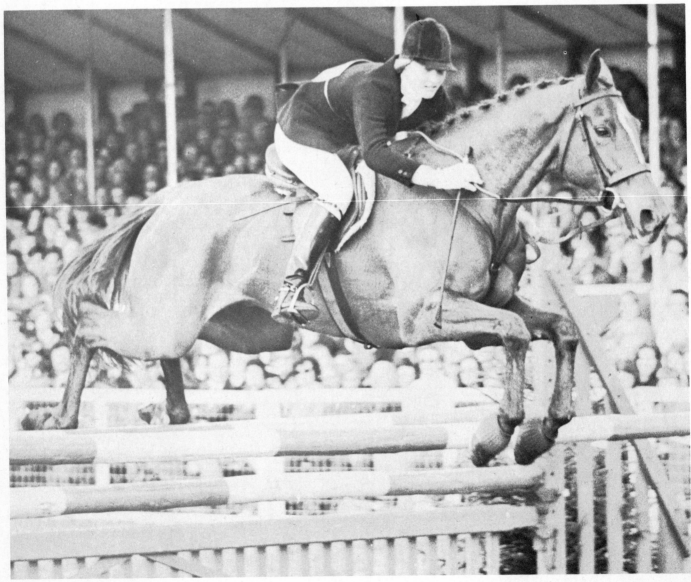

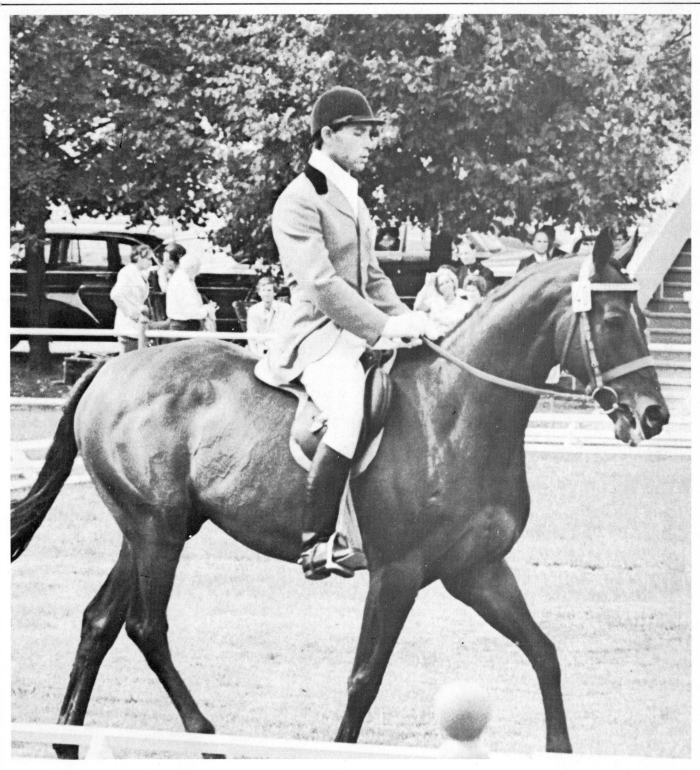

She was also the European Champion, winning the title at Copenhagen in 1957, and the first rider to win over the testing Badminton course three times. She was at the top of her sport with everything going for her, but in 1959, just three years after making the headlines, Sheila disappeared from the equestrian scene.

Her career seemed to be over. She had no top-class horse and personal problems also prevented thoughts of a return to the arena. Instead she started training horses and writing articles for equestrian magazines. In 1963 she made her comeback with a bay horse called Glenamoy. She won Little Badminton (a novice version of the big event), then finished third in the great Badminton event in 1964 and was short-listed for the Tokyo Olympic team. In the early days of Olympic three-day eventing, the Olympic rules barred women riders. It was largely due to Sheila's outstanding success in the sport that the rules were eventually changed.

Glenamoy's career was short, but Sheila produced another young horse. This time it was the small but strong Fair and Square. Sheila thought

Dressage, though often neglected by the spectator for the more spectacular cross-country phase, plays an integral part in the complete event. **Above** *A. Yevdokimov of the USSR and the 1973 European Champion goes through his paces.*

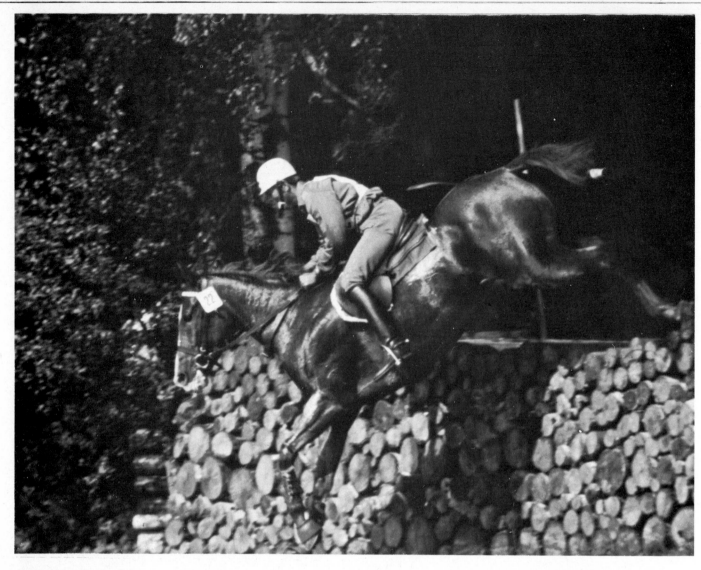

Above *A perfect landing after an extremely difficult jump by Ferdinand Croy of Austria on Etruska.*

Opposite page *Captain Mark Phillips on the Queen's horse, Columbus. In the lead after the second day of the 1974 Burghley trials he was forced to retire through injuries to the horse.*

he was to be her Olympic horse. They won the important three-day event at Burghley, Lincolnshire in the autumn of 1968. On this form, Sheila was short-listed to go to the Mexico Olympics, although she did not make the team. At Badminton in 1969, Fair and Square over-reached and broke down while negotiating a drop-fence known as Huntsman's Close. The tough little horse stumbled on, only to fall again at the next fence. This time he did not get up. His injuries were fatal.

Sheila was still determined to stay in the sport to which she was dedicated and at the Ascot Sales in 1970, she bought a thoroughbred brown gelding which had won a steeplechase at one of the minor English tracks. This one was called Here and Now. Many of the collecting-ring experts, and Sheila herself, thought that here at last she had the sort of material that matched her talent.

But the fates disagreed with them and in 1971 they dealt Sheila the most cruel blow of all. While riding in an event at Tidworth in Hampshire in the May 1971 Sheila had a crashing fall. She had crushed two vertebrae and was paralysed for some time. However, once again she has picked up the pieces of her career and she is a

much sought-after trainer and judge.

The Rome Olympics

In 1960, 73 riders from 19 nations arrived in Rome for the Olympics, where the cross-country course was one of the toughest and most sensational ever seen. One fence consisted of huge concrete drain pipes stacked up in a pyramid. Many people considered this as impossible to jump. But many riders and horses did manage it, although a few came to grief. The 'Drain Pipes' fence, as it came to be called, caused most of the trouble, but 41 of the runners finished the course, a very high percentage for a contest of this importance.

In the same Olympics one of the finest event teams ever seen arrived on the stage. This was the Gold-winning Australian team of Laurie Morgan, Neale Lavis and Bill Roycroft, riding Salad Days, Mirrabooka and Our Solo respectively. The Australians are natural horsemen. Tall, lean and hard, they believe in giving their horses as much freedom as they can, and in getting them fit to run and jump with great vigour and alacrity.

Laurie Morgan and Bill Roycroft came to England after the Olympics, enjoying some rac-

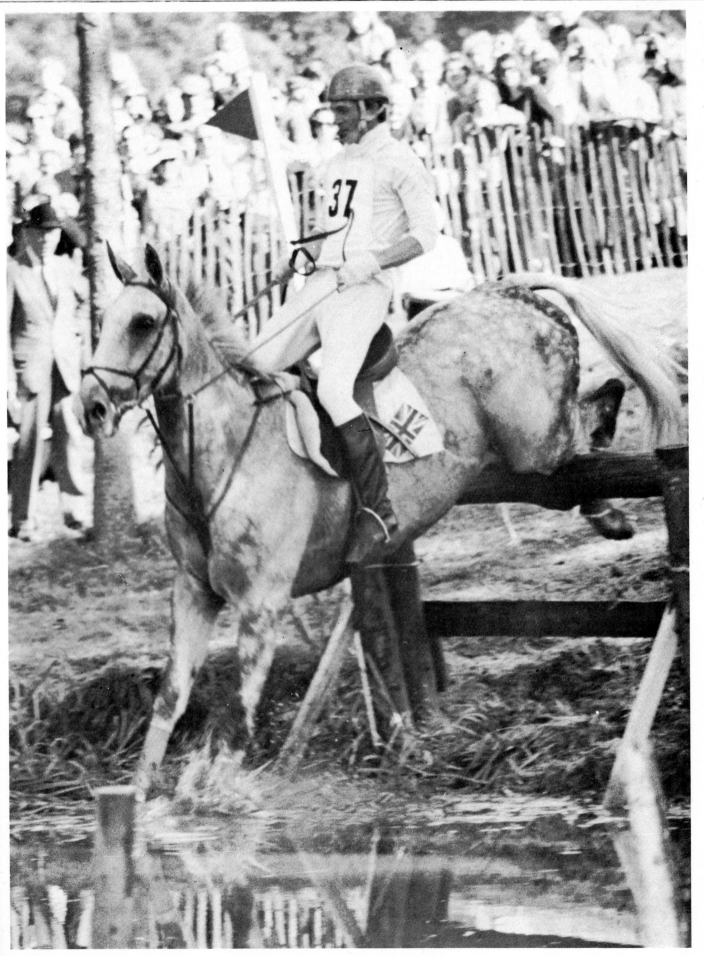

ing and show-jumping. The highlight of their stay was a win each at Badminton. In 1960, Bill Roycroft riding his Olympic horse Our Solo, and in 1961 Laurie Morgan on his Olympic horse Salad Days won the successive Badminton Trials. One of the most famous and versatile eventers ever, Salad Days was perhaps not quite as versatile as his sporting farmer-owner. In the same year that he conquered Badminton, Olympic individual gold-medallist Laurie conquered the most famous jumping track of all, Aintree. He ran out a clear winner on Colledge Master in the Foxhunter Steeplechase, run over the Grand National course and considered by many amateur riders to be more important than the Grand National itself.

Versatility is the trade-mark of Australian riders and their wiry, strong horses. Laurie Morgan's fellow-team member Bill Roycroft was not only a medal-winning event-rider and Badminton specialist, but also an Olympic show-jumping rider and a successful race rider. His most famous horse, Stoney Crossing, was placed at Badminton, a winner in the show-ring besides being a useful racehorse. He once finished third to the legendary Arkle in the Cheltenham Gold Cup. Bill, whose career spans some 40 years of competitive riding considered Stoney Crossing to be his finest horse. In 1969, he received the OBE from Queen Elizabeth II in recognition of his outstanding services to equestrian sport.

Below *In rather a flamboyant style the Russian Paul Deyev takes the water spread.*

Mexico 1968

The history of eventing is full of stories of men, women and horses battling against injury and the elements, but the 49 riders who turned out for the Mexico Olympics in 1968 must hold the record for determination in the face of adversity. In a monsoon-type storm, the British team, led by the 54-year-old Major Derek Allhusen, took the Gold medal, with the American team second and the Australians third.

In the British team at Mexico was Richard Meade on Cornishman V, and it was this horse that was to carry the diminutive Mary Gordon-Watson to fame. Cornishman is one of the best event horses ever produced in England, and he and Mary won the individual European Championship at the Haras du Pin, Normandy, France in 1969. The following year, in heavy mud and pouring rain, Mary and the free-galloping Cornishman helped England win the World Championships at Punchestown, Ireland, as well as becoming individual World title-holders in their own right. At the Munich Games in 1972, the Gold once again went to the British, and in the Olympic side this time were Mary and the great Cornishman. In the same year Richard Meade, now one of the country's leading exponents of the sport, took the individual Gold Medal on Lochinvar.

It is surprising that Ireland, one of the most famous and traditional of horse-breeding nations,

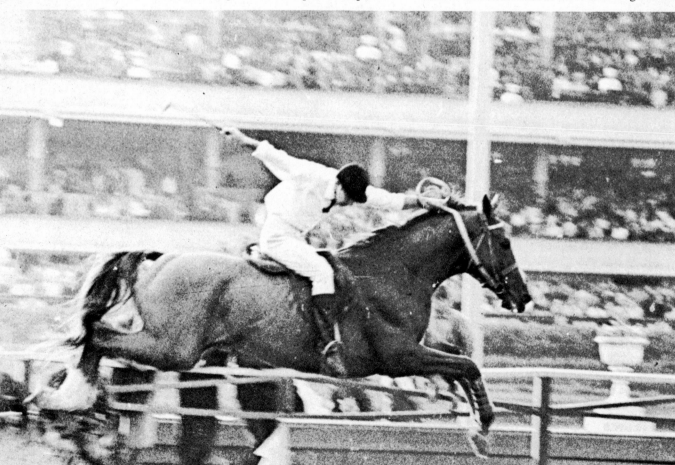

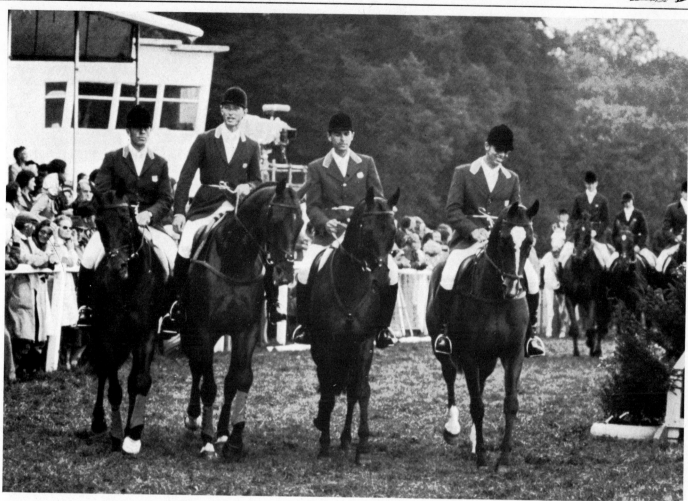

has never won an Olympic medal. This has not been through lack of trying. At the now notorious Rome Games, the Irish team, with a Silver within their grasp, were riding like demons. Several of their riders fell and remounted, one despite an injury. And Captain Harry Freeman-Jackson who three years later won Burghley on St Finbarr was collecting many points for his country. Then in the show-jumping, the final phase, he went the wrong side of a marker-flag and the entire team was eliminated.

Although three-day eventing is a young sport compared to other equestrian competitions, its short history does not lack for stories of great moments of bravery, disaster and glory. The final outstanding success story of the American team and the present World Champion, Bruce Davidson is one such moment. Their trainer Jack Le Goff, a member of the French Olympic team which took the Bronze at the 1960 Rome Olympics, worked hard and patiently to build a world-class team. They finished second at the 1968 Mexico Olympics and second again at the Munich Games in 1972. But at Burghley in 1974 they won the team World Three-Day Event Championships and the individual Gold medal. The American team comprised of Michael Plumb, veteran of three Olympic campaigns and winner of two Pan-American Golds, on Good Mixture; Bruce Davidson from Westport, Massachusetts

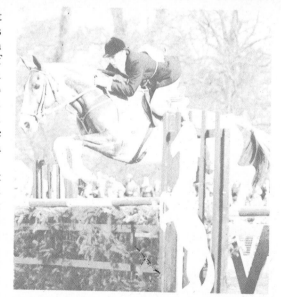

Above In 1974, the powerful American team arrived in Europe and took both the team World Championship and the individual Gold medal.

Left Precision of style marks this young rider as he takes his beautiful skewbald horse over a jump during the third day's jumping event.

with Irish Capp; ex-schoolmaster Edwin 'Denny' Emerson riding Victor Dakin; and Don Sachey from Long Island on Plain Sailing. This team not only beat the world's best on their way to the team and individual titles, but they also took the runner-up ribbons. The 24-year-old Bruce Davidson, who started riding working ponies at the age of six, is the 1974 World Champion with one of America's best-known event riders, Michael Plumb, as understudy.

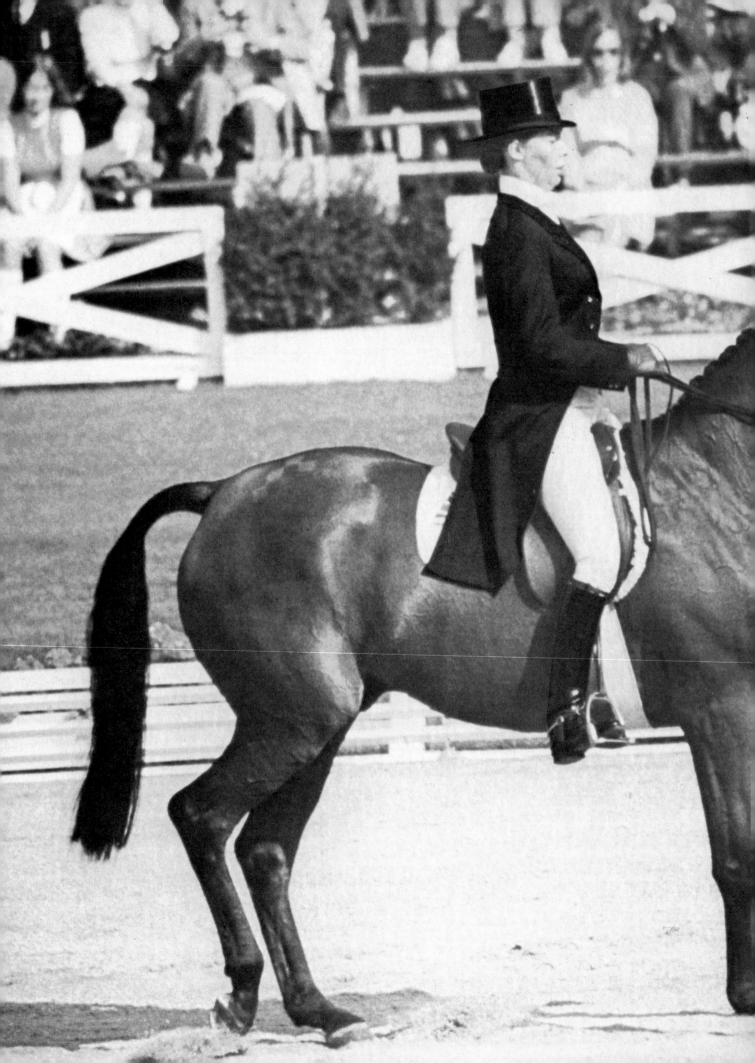

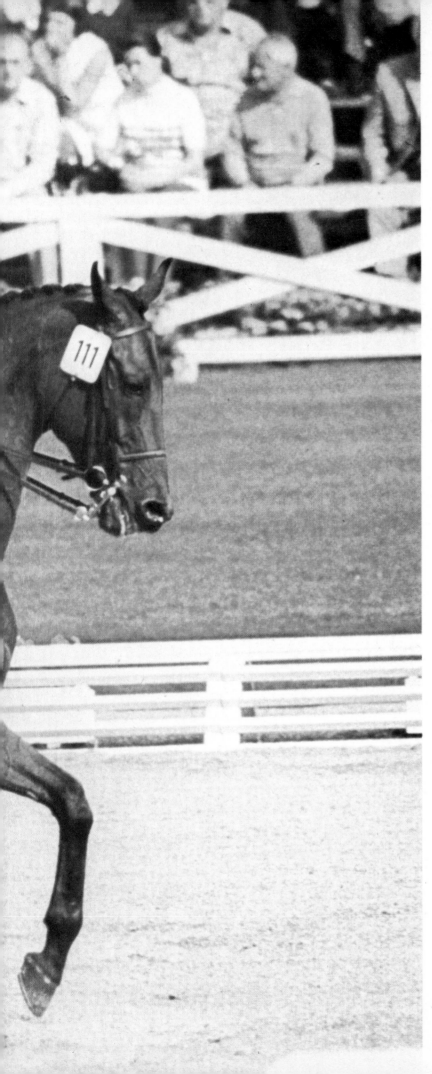

Dressage–
equitation as an art

With the Renaissance, culture and the arts returned to the classicism of the ancient civilizations. Architecture and sculpture reflected this rebirth with equestrian statues of famous men riding stylized horses. The slim, light rider of the old world gave way to the high-booted scientific equestrian, the well-fed New European with his layers of tailored clothes, his huge, luxurious saddles and his ornate stirrup-irons. The traditions of natural horsemanship, unwritten secrets handed down from father to son, were abandoned. The new sophisticates went back to the teachings of the classical horsemasters of the ancient world, where the horse and the art of riding him were the social badge of an officer and a gentleman.

Civilized 16th century man was a creature of elegance. He appreciated and understood fine music, great art and history that he could study. The chivalrous cavalryman, with his muscular, thickset mount began to rediscover the skills of horsemanship. Riding became the amusement of kings and royals and aristocrats warmed to the cry of the hounds in the great forests of Europe.

With the emergence of new techniques in the old crafts of saddlery and farriery, the riding master came to the fore with his new 'Science of Riding'. Books and papers on the techniques of the fashionable, newly-evolved science of equitation, and the training of the horse, sold in their thousands. Up to now, the subject had not been too complicated. Riding and horsemanship were naturally concentrated on hunting and warfare. Nobody required the horse to do much more than start, run fast and stop. Then, as equitation became an art, movements entered the realm of the sophisticated.

Advocate of brute force

From Italy, Federico Grisone, a 16th century royal riding master, became the father of 'artificial' equitation. Grisone did not agree with the 'kindness and co-operation' method. He blatantly advocated the use of sheer brute force in the training of the horse. Word of his teachings spread throughout the courts of Europe and England. Displays of scientific riding were given, generally in a laid-down manège. The Neapolitan School for the Training of the Cheval d'Ecole and the Cheval de Guerre was formed from Grisone's inspiration and methods.

Jennifer Loriston-Clarke takes Kadett through his paces during the individual dressage in the 1972 Munich Olympic Games.

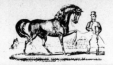

Below *Breaking through the years of domination by the Germans, the Russian team took the Olympic Gold medal in the 1972 Games.* **Right** *Elena Petushkova took the individual silver medal on Pepel.* **Left** *Ivan Kalita, a leading member of this very successful team.*

The Neapolitan School

The Neapolitan School, with its first offshoot, the Spanish School, became the most generally-accepted system of riding and training. They rode strong, short-set, far from fleet-footed, horses. These horses of entertainment and 'men-o'-war' must have been patient and docile creatures. They performed intricate 'school' movements, on the ground and in the air, under the direction of powerfully-curbed bits and long, sharp spurs. They were tied up between pillars, sometimes mounted, sometimes unridden, and physically forced to arch their necks and increase the activity of their hind-legs.

Many famous riding masters followed in the footsteps of Federico Grisone, continuing and developing his teachings. Some of them, like the famous Pignatelli, even became directors of the Neapolitan School. Others, such as James Fillis, Thomas Blundevill and the Duke of Newcastle passed the techniques to other countries.

William Cavendish, Duke of Newcastle (1592–1676) was an ardent royalist who, during a period of exile, established a famous riding school at Antwerp and published his first work on horsemanship. With the Restoration, he returned to his homeland, accepted a dukedom, and retired from public life to devote the rest of his days to his estates and the training of horses. Horsemanship may owe much to this man, but his methods and teachings are difficult to understand if it is accepted that equitation is an art. Riding in the 16th and 17th centuries was mainly governed by fashion. Fanciful illustrations in Cavendish's books show him using the same long-cheeked bits and stiff-legged, rowel-spurred style as Grisone. His horses were of the stubby, cold-blooded type (breeds as such did not exist) and if the Duke had tried some of his methods and equipment on a lighter, better-bred or more spirited horse, his high-school movements in the air would undoubtedly have been sensational to see.

Correction and reward

In 1666, a book appeared that was to be the cornerstone of the true modern art of equitation. The author was a young Frenchman called Antoine de Pluvinel. Riding instructor to Louis

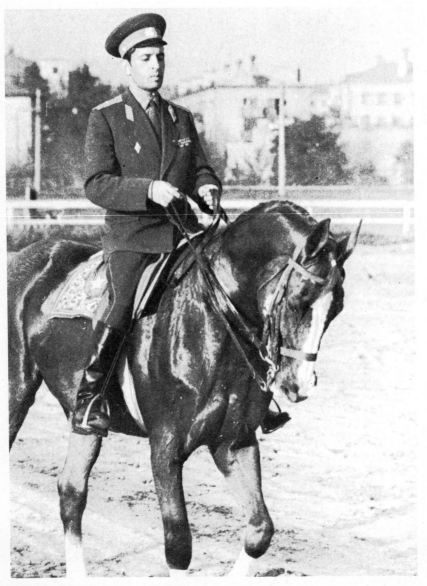

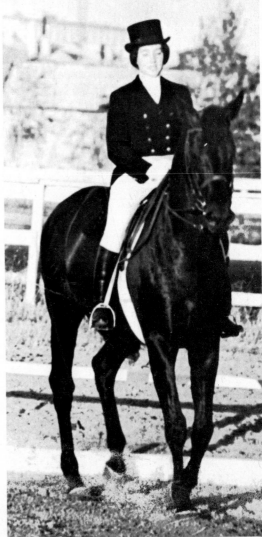

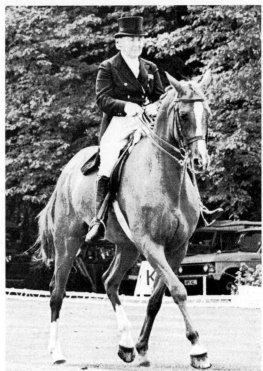

XIII, he presented his book in the style of a conversation between himself and his royal employer. De Pluvinel gave much space and thought to the notion of 'kindness and co-operation' but he went just that little bit further and insisted that, although this principle was the basis of good riding, it was all really a matter of reward and correction. Although Monsieur still followed fashion and used excessively restricting bits, at least he tried to encourage horsemen to think about the natural assets of the horse's personality. De Pluvinel's ideas were strongly frowned-upon by the purists but, with the backing of Louis XIII, his message got across to one person at least, for the crusade was taken up by Monsieur de la Guerinière another well-known horse trainer.

One of the last great directors of a riding school at Naples, de la Guerinière was the first man to state that all horses, no matter what their job is going to be, should be given basic training in obedience and flexibility. His teaching is firmly rooted in reward and correction but he adds the vital ingredients of time and patience. His ideas are the foundation-stone of what we now call dressage—not a show—but proof of suppleness and discipline.

Invisible signals and aids

Dressage in the modern sense is the basis of all equitation. Whether the horse is going to be a jumper, a hunter or just an ordinary riding horse, some form of dressage-training must be given to encourage the horse to carry a rider in a balanced and comfortable manner.

The rider controls the horse through a system of signals, known as aids, and it is by the application of these, and the horse's understanding of them, that the whole performance is turned into

a picture of elegance and grace. The natural aids at the rider's command are his hands, legs, seat and voice. In the early days of training, the rider uses his voice all the time to encourage and calm the horse. But once they enter the arena of competition the voice can no longer be used. Patience and hard work are the secret of success in this sport. It can take six years, or longer, to make a dressage horse of world class. The aids must be delicate, almost invisible, and the horse must go freely forward without losing his balance or natural spirit. Some horses, particularly male thoroughbreds, are 'naturals' at this. For them, it is a display of their superiority over other members of the herd.

Dressage has another basic but important function. The wild horse undergoes many physical changes during his lifetime. He begins as a timid foal running with his mother. Then, as he goes out into the world on his own, he develops into a gangling, inquisitive two-year-old. As life becomes a more responsible affair, he moves around a great deal, looking for rich pastures. He covers great distances, sometimes galloping, sometimes making quick changes of direction to avoid danger, sometimes playing with the others. As he follows the seasons, he finds the most nutritious food and his body begins to develop. It becomes more muscular, more powerful. His neck becomes thicker, his legs stronger and his mind sharper. From a timid foal that wobbled as he moved, he becomes an adult stallion, fast and proud. The domesticated horse develops as does his wild brother, but for him it is man and not nature who will determine his growth and development. This is one of the objects of dressage: to substitute a system of training that will bring the horse to physical and mental maturity as nature does with the wild horse of the prairies or the wind-swept steppes.

Championship Competition

Dressage, once the mysterious art of the classical schools, is now part of the Olympic Games. It has its own 'Derby' at Hickstead in England, and at Hamburg, West Germany. Each year, riders converge on these two points from all over the world. Competition is fierce while the material rewards are negligible. Now and again, someone may sell a dressage horse, usually a Grand Prix champion, for a lot of money but this is very rare. Dressage people spend a great deal of time 'making' their horses, so once they have reached international level they are loathe to part with them.

A Grand Prix or championship competition is long and complicated. There are movements on the turn, on the circle, on the straight line, at all the natural paces. The rider is also asked to show his horse at the extended paces. In dressage, 'extended' does not mean going faster, as it does in racing. It means the extension of the stride without loss of balance and without quickening. Examples of this are the 'extended walk' and

Left *One of the great characters from the dressage ring, Mrs Lorna Johnstone on El Farruco.*

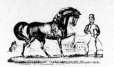

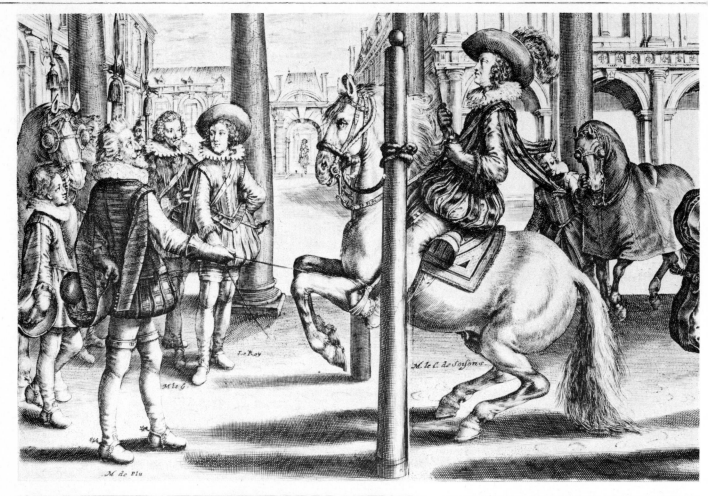

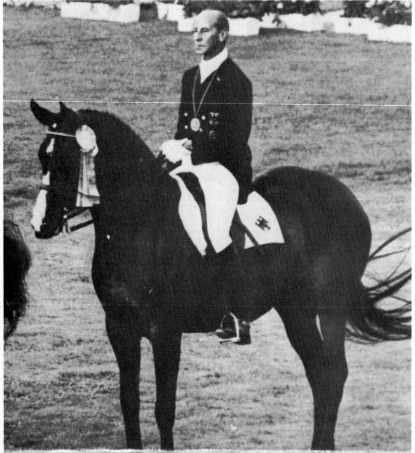

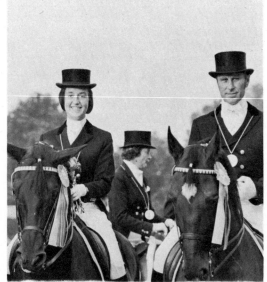

'extended trot'. In the transitions from one pace to another, the horse will be asked to lead with a certain front leg. So in cantering to the left, the horse leads with near-fore and near-hind, which means that this side of his body will be taking the slightly longer stride, thus helping his balance. Then again, the test will call for a 'counter-canter' to demonstrate the horse's obedience. This requires the horse to canter on the 'wrong' lead, as it were: for instance, when cantering to the left he will lead with the off-fore and off-hind.

As the competition builds up, more sensational movements come into the programme. The pirouette, the half-pirouette, the rein-back, the half-pass to the right and left, the piaffe where the horse remains stationary yet his limbs are moving, ready to obey the rider instantly and move off at any moment, and the passage. The passage is one of the most elegant movements the dressage-horse is asked to execute. It is similar to the gait of the trot, but the horse holds each leg in suspension much longer. It gives the impression of the animal bouncing on each beat of his stride.

The judges mark each movement for accuracy of execution. In other words, a circle must be a good circle, and if the rider asks for an extension and the horse replies with a change of pace or direction, then the markings will not be high. Also, the judges award points for the general picture of the performance: the willingness shown by the horse or the stillness or sympathy shown by the rider. In the world of really top-flight dressage riders, the 'barrier' to be crossed to enter the really top league is 1500 points. Any rider who can get into the 1500-plus bracket is at Olympic level and a world-class performer.

More a Continental sport than an Anglo-American one, the following for dressage is increasing each year and, although still a minority sport, some of the riders and horses, particularly at Grand Prix level, are beginning to emerge with more publicity. People are taking more and more interest in the art of classical equitation and this has led to an enthusiastic understanding of dressage, its demands and its execution.

The German dominance
In Germany, where there are more leading exponents than perhaps anywhere in the world, the man who draws the crowd is Dr Josef Neckermann. Ex-World Champion and winner of an Olympic Gold at the 1964 Tokyo Games on his magnificent grey horse Mariano, Josef Neckermann is the master of his art, tall and distinguished looking, with the quiet manner and confidence that men tend to get when working to such a high pitch of performance. At the International Dressage Show at Aachen, Germany in 1974, he thrilled the crowds with his fluency of movement and accuracy of figures. On that occasion, he was riding a ten-year-old, Hanoverian-bred horse called Adriano II.

The 1974 World Champion is also a German. At Copenhagen, Dr Reine Klimke on Mehmed beat Frau Lisenhoff on her Olympic mount Piaf, in an exciting 'ride-off' for the title. Third was ex-World Champion and member of the winning Russian team at Mexico, attractive Elena Petouchkova on Pepel. Fourth was another German, Harry Boldt riding Golo. These results illustrate the dominance of German riders in the sport today. However, many other nations are now taking an interest in this, the finest of equestrian events, and are now challenging this dominance.

Dressage in England
England has produced several good dressage riders since World War II: Mrs V D Williams and her well-known grey horse Little Model, Mrs Jo Hall and the very successful Mrs Lorna Johnstone. But the best-known rider of the sport in England at the moment is Mrs Jennie Loriston-Clarke and her spirited bay horse Kadett. Jennie is a beautiful rider to watch and Kadett seems to enjoy the intricate movements of the dressage test. He puts great activity into his work and holds his head in a proud and almost cocky manner. These two are just reaching world-class level. At the Aachen Show of 1974 they ran up seventh in the Grand Prix to Josef Neckermann. The impressive thing about that performance was that Jennie and Kadett broke through the magical '1500' line to finish with 1501 points. It is not often that an English rider achieves this standard in such company. And Kadett is still young as a dressage horse, so this bodes well for the future of dressage in Britain.

Dressage in the United States
In the American equestrian world, dressage is gaining more and more impetus. Whereas the Continental goes for the heavier, native-bred horse, the Americans and the English still prefer the lighter thoroughbred or thoroughbred-type horse for the sport. Leading lights in the game in the United States are Sidley Payne with his 15-year-old brown horse Felix, who gave one of their finest performances in the international arena when finishing 12th at Aachen; Elizabeth Lewis with her ten-year-old Abraxas and her Holstein Ludmilla; and Dr Lois Stephens with the Swedish-bred horse Gaspano. John Winnett and Mario, and Edith Master with her Hanoverian Sergeant, are also well-known on the international circuit, where they are putting in great performances against the best dressage riders in the world.

Reminder of heritage
The Continental has remained the master of the art of dressage, and is known for his expertise throughout the world. As a sport dressage riding is changing, but it is unique in that it still has a 'living' example of the art as it was practised in days gone by in the Spanish Riding School in Vienna.

This galleried and chandeliered academy uses and breeds the Lippizan horse, a unique type of small and muscular animal whose long and intensive training is based on the principles of the classical school of riding: that the rider should completely dominate the horse and discipline him to perform complicated movements. There is no galloping or jumping in the curriculum. Their displays are nearer to Haute-Ecole than to pure dressage, but nevertheless, the School's existence is important as a reminder of the sport's heritage, and of the perfection which the horse and rider can achieve when working together.

Flat racing –
the sport of kings or pastime of the devil?

The basic concept of horse racing has undergone virtually no change over many centuries. From a primitive contest of stamina and speed between two horses, it has developed into a colourful spectacle involving a large number of horses, bright costumes, rigidly defined rules, sophisticated electronic equipment and sometimes fantastic sums of money. But the essential feature has always been the same—the horse that finishes first is the winner.

From the ramparts of classical riding, the jockey and the stable lad are looked down upon as rather poor examples of the equestrian rider. True enough, the jockey may not know much about performing a carefully-executed half-pass across the paddock. Equally, the jockey may not mount according to the strictest principles of some dressage manual. Instead, with one spring, he can vault into the saddle and let his horse walk away on a free rein. Freedom is the magic of racing, thoroughbreds galloping across plains are its glamour, but the reality is a young stable lad riding out at dawn, perched on a fit, hot-blooded horse.

The origins of organized racing

A world of cigar smoke, and of fortunes won and lost, is the back-drop to one of the oldest equestrian sports—flat-racing. The Greeks staged a form of flat-racing at the original Olympiad, with young boys sitting bare-back on large horses, galloping at great speeds round a track. The racing of horses was popular in ancient Persia, Arabia and Egypt. No accurate records have been found but it seems, rather like the early Olympiads, that this was merely some form of mounted games.

The real start of organized racing was in the England of James I. James was not a very good rider and the winning post did not see his Royal colours flashing past very often. But his interest was a great boon to the history of racing for in an attempt to improve the quality of his luckless string of running horses he imported the first 'Eastern' stallion into England.

Racing is a game of luck, a gambler's business, but King James' stallion from Constantinople did not bring the radical change and miracle that he wished. His injection of hot-blood into the veins of the native horses of the Royal stables failed to produce either luck or fortune. But it started a trend and others picked up the idea, far more successfully, of trying to breed a perfect racing machine—a true thoroughbred.

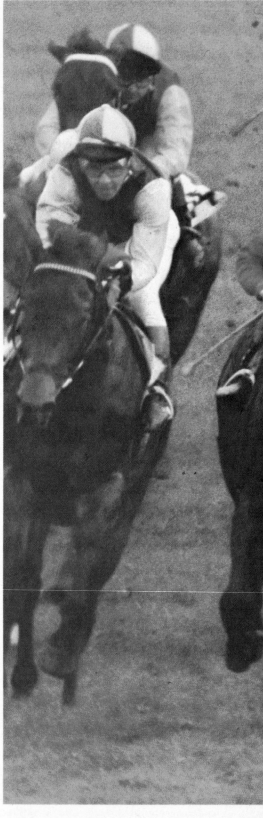

Racing already existed in impromptu forms and took place mainly at local fairs. Dealers ran races for wagers and boys, as the jargon went at the time 'did ride upon horses with the desire for praise and hope of victory'. The landed gentry enjoyed nothing more than a sizeable bet on a match between two well-known local horses. The jockeys were grooms from the hunt stables or

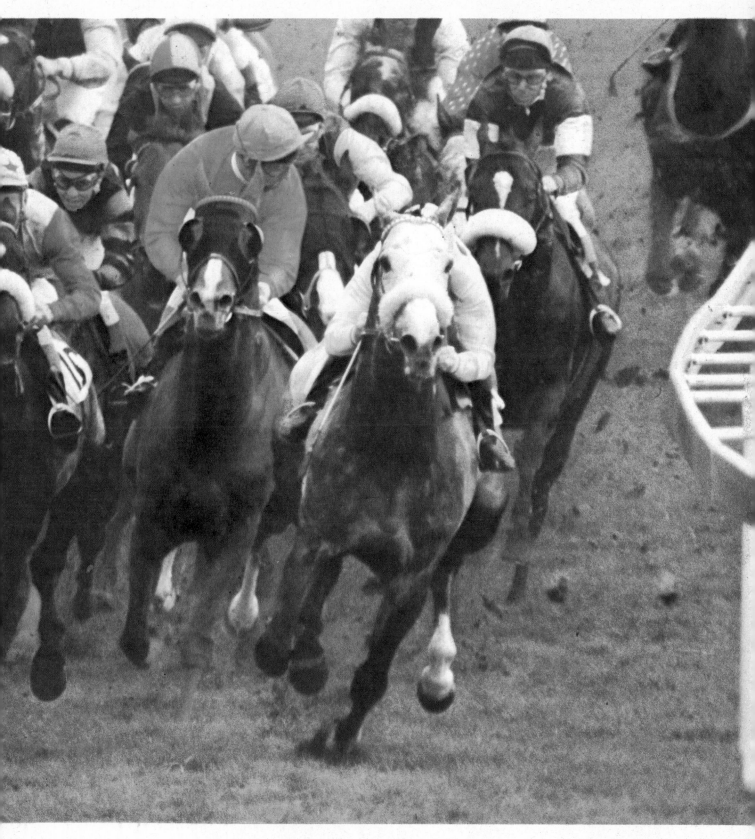

dealers' yards. The tracks were from one land-mark to another, and the rules were made up for individual races. It was all fairly disorganized with no generally recognized rules and no governing body, but with plenty of enjoyment. The ill-fated Charles I established the first Royal Stud and had 139 horses at the time of his death. But the Protectorate frowned upon racing, and what

little development there was subsequently disappeared, or carried on discreetly, if not secretly, until the reign of Charles II.

The three Arab stallions
The year 1660 was that of the Restoration, the crowning of Charles II, known as 'the father of the British turf'. Charles loved racing, and rode

Running neck and neck as they race round the final bend and head for home. The jockey needs to rely on all his skill and tenacity to to be able to pull ahead of his rivals and win in such an overcrowded situation.

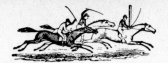

in several races himself, surely the only English reigning monarch to be a flat-race jockey. Where James failed, Charles succeeded. He was a successful breeder, owner and jockey. He created the Round Course and started some form of organized system at Newmarket, a favourite haunt of the luckless James. He was a great patron of the turf and set up Kings Plates, prizes of silver cups and money, to be run for among competitive riders.

The importation of 'Eastern' stallions gathered impetus under his reign and three of these in particular have entered the record books as the creators of the 'racehorse'. These were the Byerley Turk, the Darley Arabian and the Godolphin Arabian. This trio was mated with the already established native mares and the end-product was the warm-blooded thoroughbred: a racing machine capable of making his owner a small fortune in less than 60 seconds running time, and losing the same when out at exercise.

The Jockey Club

Little is known of the origins of the Jockey Club said to have started around this time. The members of this select and secret governing body are the controllers of racing in Great Britain. It is known that in 1752 the Jockey Club took charge of racing at Newmarket, built themselves a coffee room and laid down the rules of racing. These became the model for other racing countries and now jockeys can ride almost anywhere in the world with very few problems concerning the rules.

Such is the historical background to the shouting bookmakers and whistling tic-tac men of

The three Arab stallions from which every thoroughbred racehorse in the world is descended. **Right** *The Byerley Turk (from the original picture by John Wootton). According to legend he was owned by a Captain Byerley who rode him during William III's wars in Ireland.*
Below *The Godolphin Arabian (from the original picture by George Stubbs RA). Imported from Paris, where it is said he once pulled a water-cart, he eventually came into the possession of the Earl of Godolphin.*
Below right *The Darley Arabian (from the original picture by John Wootton) – the dominant ancestor of the modern flat racing stock.*

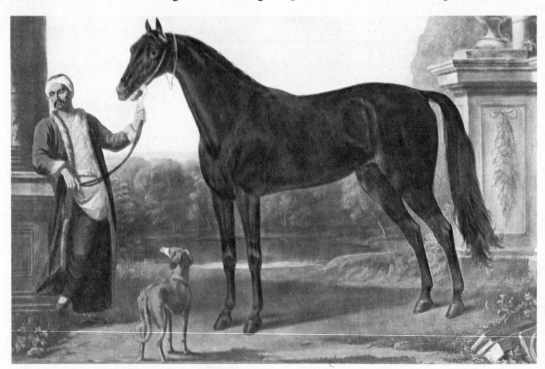

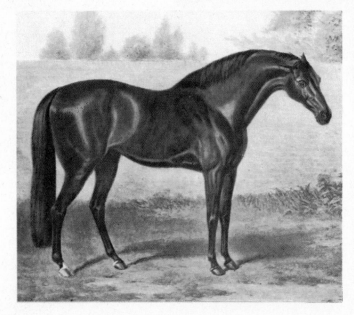

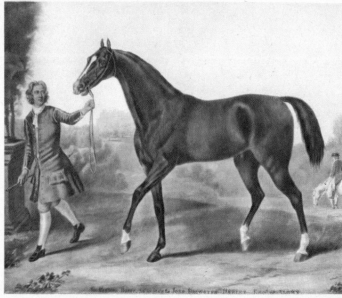

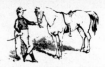

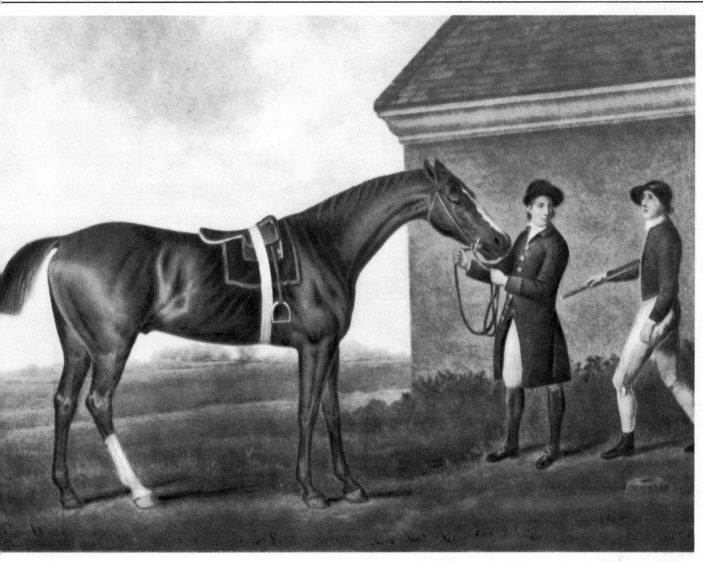

today. The horses of that time are the ancestors of the famous colours now known on every race-course in the world. The racing set-up of the time of Charles II forms the basic traditions of the feudal, close-knit circle that is now the inner core of the sport—trainers, jockeys, stable lads and the thoroughbred horse.

'Eclipse first, the rest nowhere'

Flying Childers was the first famous 'match winner' of racing history. But the most famous horse of the 18th century was a colt bred by the Duke of Cumberland in 1764 and christened Eclipse. Few names in racing history are as well-known. He was sired by Marske out of a mare known as Spilletta and raced in the colours of Mr William Wildman and Colonel Dennis O'Kelly. Eclipse did not start racing until he was five-years-old. His first race was in May 1769 and in his short career he was never beaten on the turf and never touched with the whip. He retired to stud in the autumn of 1771. Only one horse ever gave Eclipse a real race and it is said that Bucephalus never recovered from the effort. The saying of the day was: 'Eclipse first, the rest nowhere'. He was without doubt the greatest racehorse of his

century. His influence on the breeding of future racehorses can be seen in the record books. Over 100 of his descendants have won the Epsom Derby.

Early races

The riding techniques of the early jockeys came from both the classical school of riding and the hunting field. The horses were big, rangy creatures with light, straight-cut saddles and most of them raced in the traditional full double-bridle or a double-reined bridle. They were strong, highly strung animals and the jockeys were thin, wiry but tough men. They had to be. Races were run in heats so that the horses and jockeys would canter down to the starting-post, sometimes as often as four times before finally running for the winner's crown. These races were no five-furlong dashes along a lush green straight with running rails, but a punishing grind on an up-and-down track marked with flags, often with up to 6.4km (4 miles) to run in each heat. Jockeys had to be prepared to push themselves, to draw upon reserves of stamina because winning races provided the chance to earn big money. Like the prize fighter the jockey could line his pockets

Above *The great Eclipse (from a painting by George Stubbs). In 18 starts he never suffered a defeat and in 8 of these no horse could be induced to race against him. Bucephalus was the only horse ever to threaten Eclipse's unbeaten record in a race during which Bucephalus over-reached himself and had to be taken out of training.*

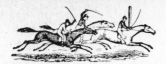

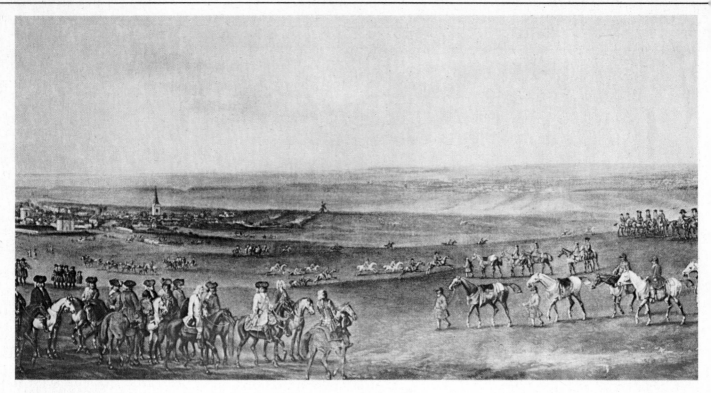

*Racing in England has had
a long association with
royalty – dating back to the
sadly unsuccessful James I.*
Above *The Hanoverian
kings were no exception.
Here George I arrives at
Newmarket in 1722.*

richly if he gave the gambling aristocrats value for money.

These early jockeys sat bolt upright in their small saddles, their legs hanging down to their natural length. The trick was to fix the running martingale (check straps) to the snaffle rein (upper rein) of the double bridle. This gave the jockey a means to check and steady his mount and to keep his head down without upsetting him. By raising his hand, he could bring the martingale into play, at the same time operating off the softest mouthpiece of the bridle. If he required more control, the lower rein, working off the weymouth of the bridle, was left free and ready to be used whenever circumstances demanded. At the start of the race, for example, where the horse might over-anticipate the starter's flag or during the race when a change of position or line might be forced on the race rider the lower rein was used. For difficult rides they changed the system round, putting the running martingale on the lower, more severe rein, to give a two-way leverage on the animal's mouth.

One reason for putting a man on a racehorse's back is to encourage the creature to run faster than he would on his own. Some horses, particularly colts, will, without assistance, run faster than fellow members of the pack. Other horses would need plenty of coaxing. When a thoroughbred runs he flattens and lengthens his body, getting closer to the ground while stretching his head and neck out in front of him—not only poetry in motion but economy in action. The early jockey's job was to have the horse gallop as evenly as possible in this lengthened form and to do it better than the other contestants. Through the bit he could control and regulate this change of form. To back this up he carried a long whip

and wore sharp spurs.

In the 17th and 18th centuries the racing fraternity, especially the titled ones, rather liked the public image of lovers of horse racing and, above all, patrons of that noble beast, the thoroughbred. But often in those early days of the 'Sport of Kings' a horse returned to the winner's enclosure with blood running from his flanks or large throbbing weals on his quarters. Then, as now, there were two main reasons for racing horses against each other. One was to win a big wager, the other was to win classics and prestige. And when the money is down, sentiment comes a poor second.

Fred Archer

The first nationally-known race jockey hailed from Cheltenham in Gloucestershire, a traditional centre of foxhunting. This tall, moody reinsman, whose battles with the scales were tougher than his fights for the winning post, was Frederick Archer. Born in 1857, he was worshipped by some as one of the greatest jockeys, detested by others as a cruel and devious man. A rider of ice-cool nerve from the age of 13, he was to ride the winners of 2748 races from some 8004 rides in public. Many of these winners were of classic races including five Derbys, six St Legers, four 2000 Guineas, four Oaks and two 1000 Guineas. And, despite his short career, Fred Archer was champion English flat-race jockey for thirteen seasons. This record was not beaten until well into the 20th century and was no mean feat in days of uncomfortable travel, before the age of the charter aircraft connections to meetings up and down the country. A difficult and temperamental character, constant dieting and deprivation eventually affected his mind and, as

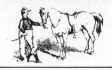

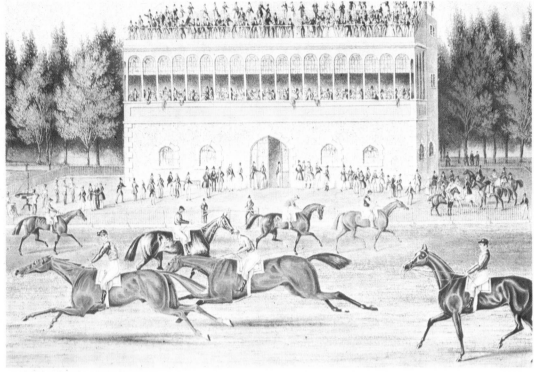

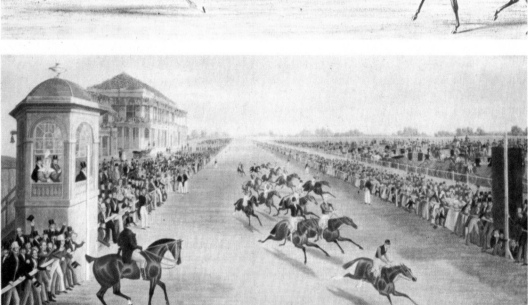

many jockeys after him were to find, the demands of his profession left him with long bouts of mental depression. It was during one of these periods that he took his own life in 1886, leaving almost £67,000 ($160,130) in his will.

Fred Archer was not a man to tangle with during a race. He rode in the scientific style, using long leathers, sitting deep seat in the saddle leaving the horse's head free so that he flattened and extended to the maximum. As far as Archer was concerned, the art of winning races lay in this technique and in the persuasive power of whalebone and steel.

The perfect racing machine

One of the most famous and successful racehorses with which the legendary Fred Archer was associated was St Simon. St Simon was sired by the 1875 Derby winner Galopin and out of a mare called St Angela, who had a very poor breeding record. After St Simon's breeder, Prince Batthyany, had died from heart failure on the steps of the Jockey Club luncheon-room at Newmarket, the Duke of Portland purchased him at the bargain price of 1600 guineas ($4015). Despite his lack of classic potential this turned out to be one of the best buys of racing history. The colt won the Ascot Gold Cup and the Goodwood Cup in 1884 and finished his racing career with an unbeaten record. St Simon was said to have electrifying acceleration and the finest race he and Archer ever ran was in the Ascot Gold Cup. In that race they beat a horse called Tristan, which had won the Gold Cup the previous year and finished second in the Grand Prix de Paris of 1881, 20 lengths behind the great American

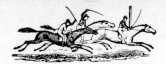

Right *Fred Archer –
champion jockey at the age
of 17, he never lost the
title in his short but
spectacular career.*

Centre top *Archer with
the great Ormonde. In his
last season Archer rode
Ormonde to victory in the
2,000 Guineas, the Derby
and St Leger.*

Far right top *George
Fordham, Archer's great
rival. Artistic and polished,
Fordham often came out
best in matched races
against Archer.*

Centre *The long striding
Kincsem who dumfounded
the punters by taking the
Goodwood Cup in 1876
after a long string of
successes on the Continent.*

Below *Fordham's only
winning mount in the
Derby, Sir Bevis, and
Wheel of Fortune, ridden
successfully by Archer in
the Oaks of the same year,
1879.*

Centre below *St Simon,
a great racehorse and even
greater sire – his progeny
won all five English classics
in 1900 and still continue to
take the top prizes even
today.*

Below far right *At 5ft
10in, Archer had a
continual weight problem.
In a bout of depression after
a period of wasting he took
his own life at the age of 29.*

horse Foxhall. Fred Archer, who had won the
Triple Crown, Derby, 2000 Guineas and St Leger
on Ormonde, always claimed that St Simon was
the greater of the two and Matt Dawson his
trainer, who produced six Derby winners, said
that St Simon was the finest horse he ever
handled.

St Simon was the real racing machine, a horse
with a perfect action and the intelligence and
temperament to go with it. As a stallion he
proved himself capable of passing these qualities
on to his progeny. He headed the list of leading
stallions no less than nine times, more often than
any other stallion had done since the 1787 Derby
winner, Sir Peter.

By the late 18th and early 19th centuries the
Jockey Club began to realize the potential of
flat-racing. They realized that they had now a
sport on their hands capable of appealing to the
popular imagination. The structure of modern
racing began to take shape. Races of varying
distances and handicaps became part of the racing
calendar. Great races like the 2000 Guineas run
at Newmarket, the Derby, first run over 1·6km
(1 mile) at Epsom and later extended to 2·4km
(1½ miles) and the St Leger were now recognized
as 'classic' races for colts. The fillies had their
own classics, such as the Oaks and the 1000
Guineas. Two-year-olds streaking along a straight
sprint track became popular with breeders and
the racing public. Bookmakers acquired a certain
respectability from the masters of the racing
game. For a gentleman to welsh on his bets was
shame indeed.

Racing on the Continent

In Europe meanwhile, horseracing had already
passed the embryo stage. The seed had been
sown by exiled English Royalist officers at the
time of Oliver Cromwell. Racing provided a way

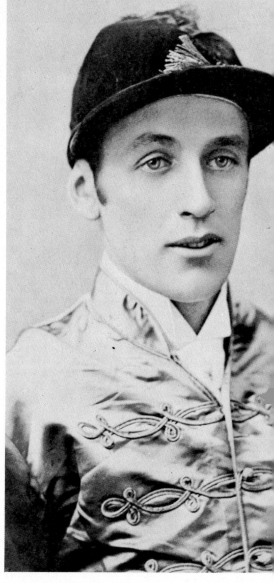

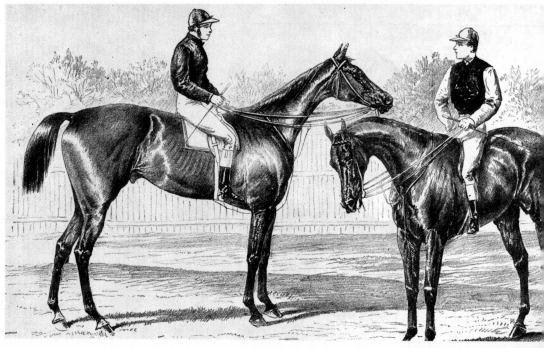

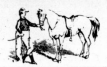

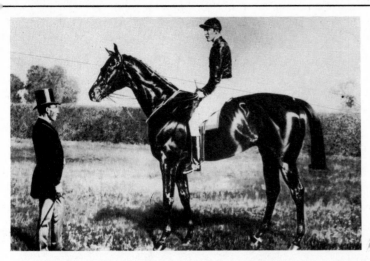

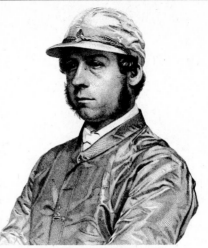

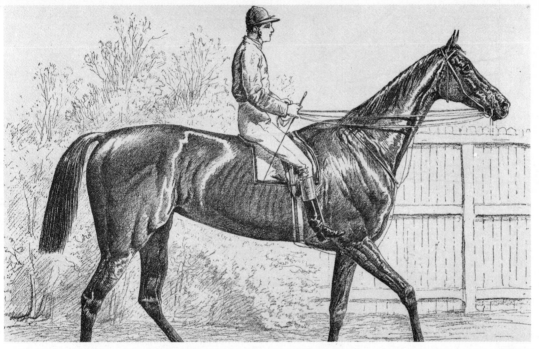

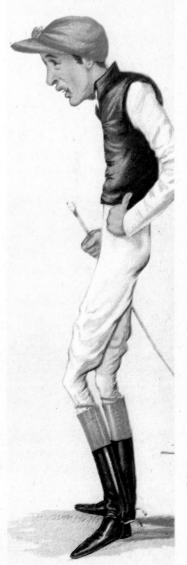

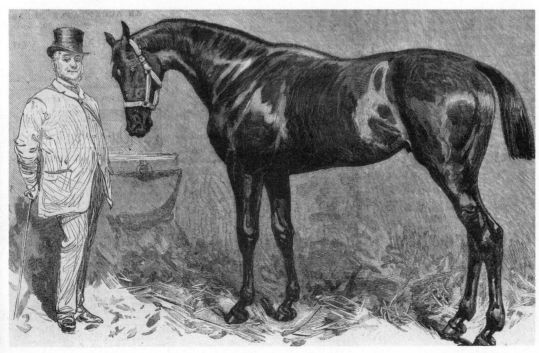

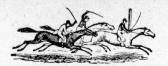

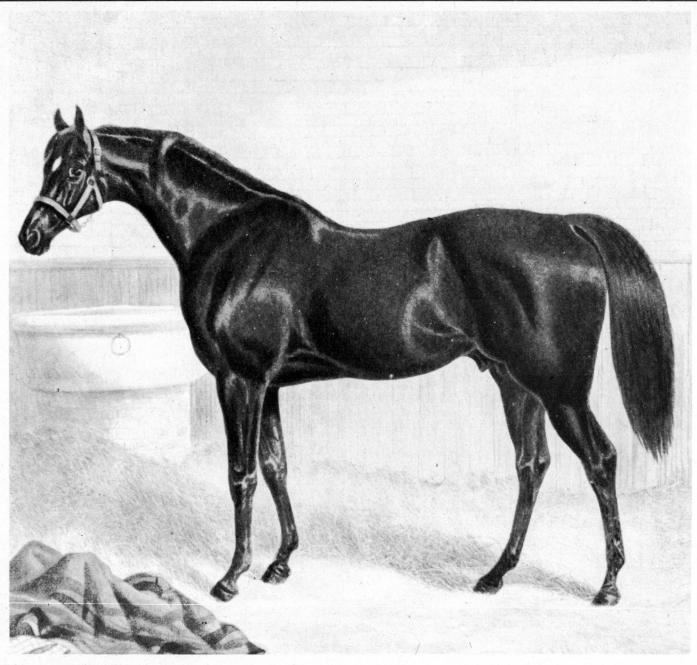

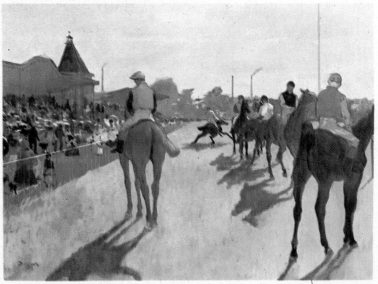

of passing the idle days in the limbo which had overtaken their lives and careers. The continental public was not much attracted by the sport but some aristocrats soon took to it. It is ironic that France, a nation which was to become one of the most influential in flat-racing, should have started off with little apparent interest in the sport. Many of the 'Eastern' stallions that contributed to or created the thoroughbred had in fact passed through France on their way to England.

From the 14th century to the latter half of the 18th century, racing in France was a very makeshift affair. Then, in 1776, the first regular course was created on the Plaine des Sablons and a committee comprising the Duc de Chartres, the Comte d'Artois and the Marquis de Conflans was convened to organize racing there. But any chance of the new sport spreading, as it was rapidly doing in England at that time, was soon

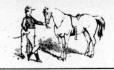

brought to a halt by the French Revolution and later by the Napoleonic Wars. French racing almost disappeared until ardent enthusiast Lord Henry Seymour decided that something should be done to bring the sport into line with its English counterpart. Lord Henry, whose father was the third Marquess of Hertford, was born in France and lived there most of his life. But, like so many Englishmen living abroad, he kept his Anglo-Saxon life-style and canvassed his influential friends for support for his idea of creating a Jockey Club. He was fortunate in having as one of his closest friends the then heir to the throne, Ferdinand Philippe, Duc d'Orleans.

Societe d'Encouragement

Their intention was to form a fashionable social club in Paris that would also, through a committee, administer racing and some form of bloodstock industry. Seymour and his friends soon splintered off from the social side of the club and formed the Société d'Encouragement pour l'Amelioration des Races de Chevaux en France. This organization, better known as the 'Société d'Encouragement' was recognized by the French government in the spring of 1834 and the first racecourse supervized by an officially-established governing body was laid out on the Champ de Mars on the left bank of the Seine river where the Eiffel Tower now stands. The opening meeting took place on Sunday, May 4, 1834.

Pur-Sang Anglais

Having established racing, the Société d'Encouragement decided to turn its attention to the breeding of fine racehorses. In the past practically no thought had been given to this side of the sport and it was decided to take advantage of the work of the English Jockey Club in this field. By importing foundation stallions and mares from England, the French breeders knew that the most they could hope for was to equal the standard on the other side of the Channel. But now with organized racing and a planned calendar it would be feasible, in generations to come, to create a French racehorse that would be as good if not better than any in the world. This dream did not really take full effect until the latter part of the 19th century. In 1834 the French Stud Book was established and the creators of the bloodstock industry in France paid their English counterparts the greatest of all compliments by decreeing that the thoroughbred in France should be known as the 'Pur-Sang Anglais'.

For the Parisian, a day at the races in the Bois de Boulogne or the Champ de Mars was a great pleasure. But soon they were to be served with an even more exotic dish. On the outskirts of Paris lay a small town with an attractive, moated Chateau, sweeping parkland and natural forest that was to become the French answer to Newmarket. Chantilly, now known as the Cité du Cheval, was the stage for the first Prix du Jockey Club, the French Derby, in 1836. At first the

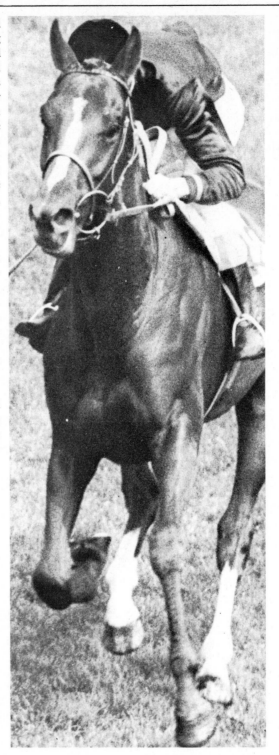

runners in all races organized by the Société had to be bred in France in order to encourage breeders. Many of the stallions imported from England were classic winners. There does not seem to have been a French equivalent of Fred Archer and no noted national jockeys emerged until the 20th century.

Racing in the United States

In America, the settlers quickly established the sports of flat-racing and trotting. The young Americans liked the spectacle and the gambling of horse racing. This ancestral home of the horse

Opposite page top *For years France lagged surprisingly behind England in the racing world. It was not until the appearance of Gladiateur that France achieved parity in race horse breeding. In 1865 Gladiateur took most of the leading prizes including the 2,000 Guineas, the Derby, the Grand Prix de Paris and the St Leger to earn himself the title 'The Avenger of Waterloo'.*

Opposite page below *By the late 19th century a day at the race course was a popular pursuit for the fashionable Parisian. This mood is reflected in the art of the period as in Degas' Chevaux des Courses shown here.*

Left *In the 20th century France has provided many winners on the major international race circuit. One of the most successful was Sea Bird who took 1965 Epsom Derby and Prix de l'Arc de Triomphe and was sent to stud in the United States at the end of the season.*

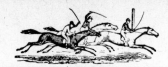

was to be the birthplace of the new race rider and the new racehorse.

The essence of progress for the pioneer American was speed. To get things done quickly was the secret of their success. The dynamic philosophy of the 'go-getters' overflowed into their sport and the stopwatch became the judge of the thoroughbred and the brain of the jockey. Tracks were designed and laid out for speed, flat and almost circular. Even now the American jockey's style is to get his horse balanced quickly, then to make him run and make him run fast.

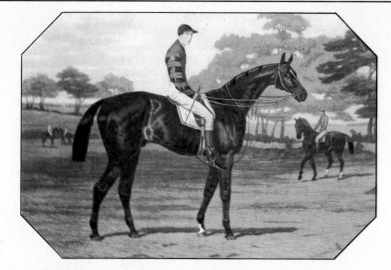

Medley and Diomed

Most sporting historians accept that the first racecourse was established by Richard Nicolls, the governor of New York, at Salisbury Plain, later known as Hempstead Plain, on Long Island. In 1665, Nicolls offered a silver cup to be run for over this course. But it was not until some years after the War of Independence that the American thoroughbred and racing became a widespread reality. At that time the enthusiasts decided to bring the form of racing, and the type of horse used, into line with the already successful English model. The English stallions imported into the country were to have the greatest influence on the bloodstock industry. These were Medley and Diomed.

Medley was nine-years-old when he arrived in Virginia, and the winner of 12 races in England. He did not win many races as a stallion but he did turn out to be a very successful producer of brood mares. Many of his daughters were mated with the unpredictable Diomed and it was this female line that played such an important part in the evolution of the American racing horse.

Diomed was owned and raced in England by that first dictator of the British turf, Sir Charles Bunbury. He won the Epsom Derby and as a three-year-old was unbeaten. He then seemed to fade rapidly and was eventually put to stud where, once again he was known as a failure. Sir Charles then sold him to John Hoomes, a Virginian breeder, for 50 guineas ($125). Diomed seemed to change in America and John Hoomes eventually passed him on for a very quick profit to Colonel Miles Selden for £1000 ($2390). Dismissed as a failure in England, Diomed produced some of the finest racetrack performers in America. He was still serving mares at the age of 29 and eventually died in 1808 at the old age of 31.

One of Diomed's most illustrious sons was Sir Archie, a 16 hands bay horse. Foaled in 1805, he was possibly the greatest racehorse of his day. He won the Jockey Club Purse at Fairfield, with great ease, took the Jockey Club Purse at Petersburg and followed this by stranding a very high-field at Halifax, North Carolina.

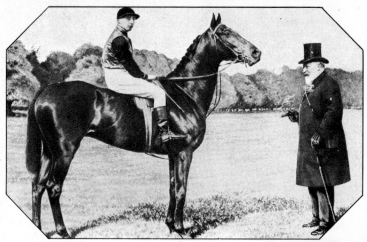

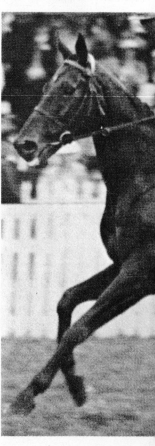

North v South

Diomed's grandson, Sir Henry, was involved in one of America's most famous races. This was run over the Union Course at New York in 1823.

His opponent was a horse called American Eclipse, named after the celebrated English horse Eclipse, and the stake was an astounding $20,000 (£8368). The race caused tremendous interest and for the 60,000 strong crowd it developed into something deeper than just a horse race. For them it was a match between North and South, with American Eclipse representing the North and Sir Henry the South.

The match was run, in what was then the classic style, of punishing 6·4km (4 miles) heats. Sir Henry won the first heat by a length—American Eclipse had been injured by the excessive use of his jockey's whip. The betting now became furious and in the second heat American Eclipse, with another jockey on board, ran out the winner by two lengths. Both horses were now beginning to show signs of fatigue from their strenuous efforts as they cantered down for the final heat. American Eclipse, also very closely related to Diomed, showed the superior stamina and won the final heat. But he took a minute longer than Sir Henry had done in the first heat.

The Kentucky Derby

Although the administrators of the American turf were influenced by the pattern created in England, they took the racing a stage further. Speed was what they looked for in racing and in 1875

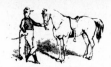

the greatest of the American classics, the Kentucky Derby, was run at Churchill Downs, Louisville over 2km (1·25 miles) as against Epsom's 2·4km (1·5 miles).

The Kentucky Derby, with the Belmont Stakes, first run at Jerome Park in 1867, and the Preakness Stakes, introduced in 1873 over the Pimlico track in Maryland, formed the American equivalent of the English 'classics' and the winner of all three gained the sought-after title of Triple Crown winner. The Belmont Stakes is now looked upon as the senior of the three contests. It moved from Jerome Park to Morris Park in 1890 until Belmont Park, opened in 1905, became its permanent home. The Preakness Stakes has had the most chequered career of the three. It was abandoned in 1890, revived four years later at Gravesend in New York and finally returned to its original home at Pimlico in 1909, where it is run in the middle of May.

The 'monkey seat'

Early racing was to be pushed into modern times by a man who, although small in stature, revolutionized the sport. This riding revolution occurred from the observations and experiments of an American called Todhunter Sloan, the inventor of the 'monkey seat'. While Fred Archer and his contemporaries were spurring home winners, Sloan began to examine riding techniques after he had watched Negro stable-lads trying to kneel on their horses in fun. But he noticed something that others did not see. The horses ran faster, more freely, and with more natural

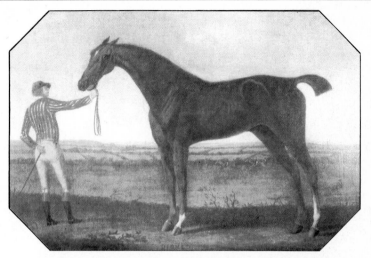

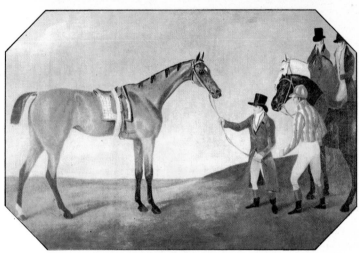

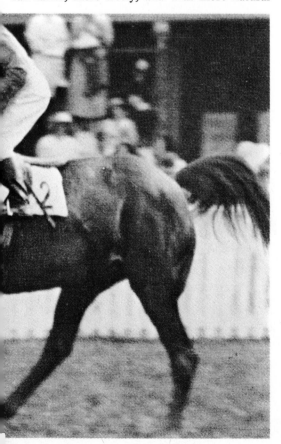

enthusiasm with the rider so mounted.

So Sloan shortened his stirrup-leathers and crouched down behind his horse's neck. He found that the horse could operate better if left to rely on his natural talent. With Sloan's techniques the rider can get behind the horse's neck and cut down the wind resistance, making the horse's job easier. With shorter leathers and a forward-cut saddle his point of balance is concentrated on the withers of his mount. There is practically no muscle movement at the gallop on this part of the horse's body (the withers are on either side of a high ridge bone at the base of the neck and just above the shoulders) so the rider interferes to the minimum and assists to the maximum. His seat can be lifted out of the saddle and off the horse's back to aid the horse's racing action. But the really clever part of this technique is that the rider's position gives leverage to the feet and body weight (by placing the feet forward or by straightening the body) so that a small lightweight can control a muscle-powered thoroughbred a hundred times stronger than himself.

Tod Sloan had no need for long spurs, as his short leathers allowed him to use the rhythm of the horse's movement to extract more speed, and to use his hands and shoulders to 'push' the horse out to his maximum extension. A whip the length of a fishing rod was no good to him either. In

Opposite page top *The first American horse to come to the fore in Britain, Iroquois, whose victory in the 1881 Epsom Derby, ridden by Fred Archer, held up business on Wall Street.*

Opposite page bottom *Minoru, the only winner of the Derby to wear the colours of a reigning monarch.*

Centre *The famous partnership of the 1920s and 30s, Donoghue on Brown Jack.*

Top *Diomed, a failure in England but a leading sire in the United States.*

Above *One of the few fillies to have won the Derby, Sir Charles Bunbury's Eleanor.*

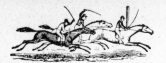

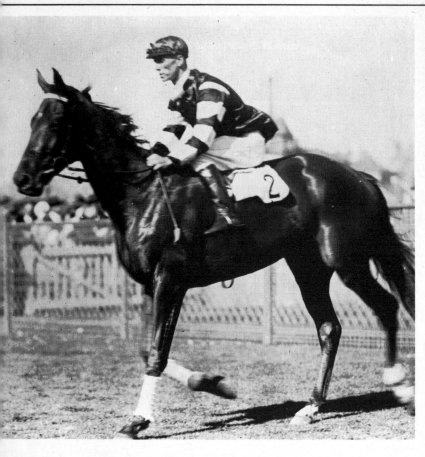

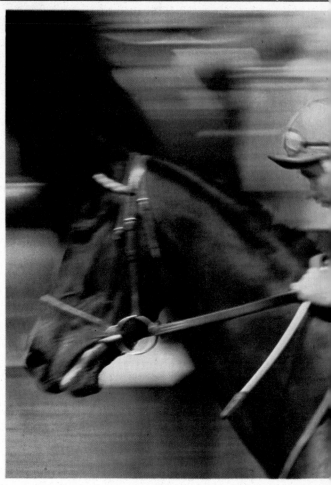

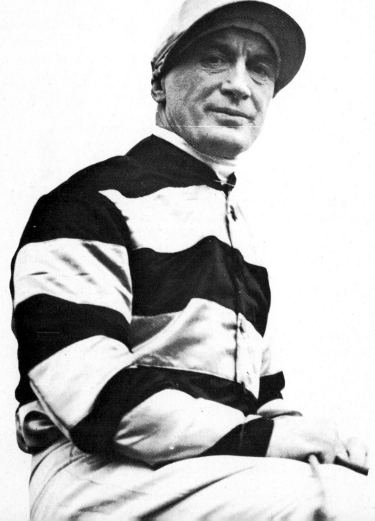

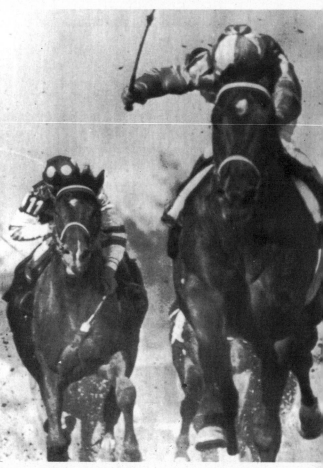

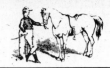

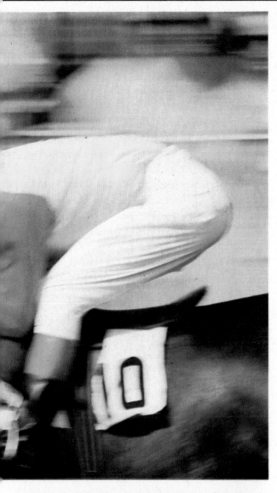

fact, in his low crouching position it would have been in his way; so he carried a shorter whip. The effort of winning then became no longer a bad memory for the racehorse.

Sloan left no reams of paper covered with technical phrases or theories, just the proof of his ideas in action and the example of success for others to follow. He was a master of the art of waiting in front and his judgement of pace was brilliant. At the peak of his career in the late 1800s he was earning $35,850 (£15,000) a year. In 1897 he brought his new style to England. As with all things revolutionary, the captains of the 'sport' frowned upon the 'monkey' seat. But Sloan astonished all with his crouching technique by riding many winners.

The Classic Era

Following Sloan's revolution, a great era of classic horses and jockeys opened up. What equestrian purists looked upon as a group of rough-necks proved themselves to be natural horsemen participating in the horse's natural talent. Unlike the military rider, the stable lad and apprentice jockey came into racing with little or no knowledge or tradition of horses, most of them from very poor backgrounds and with a limited education. Some of them had never sat on a horse or been near one before arriving at the stable yard for their first morning's work. But racing became the show business side of the equestrian world, the only section of the sport where the rags-to-riches fairy-tale could come true.

These undersized boys had a desire, a determination and a dream to ride winners. They starved for success and recognition. Competition within the trainer's yard was fierce and jealousy was the driving force that made the strong keep down the weak. In the early days of the 20th century, lightweight boys were plentiful and out of every 500 entering the game, only one would get a ride in public. One ride in public or one win in an apprentice race does not make a jockey, but it is better than never having done it.

In flat-racing history, the beginning of the 20th century reads almost like a Hollywood script, with famous jockeys being suspended, worshipped by royalty, blackmailed by bookies or adored by film stars. Fortunes changed hands quicker than the horses ran their races. Great names appeared in the record books. Brownie Carslake, one of the first of many Australian jockeys to settle and ride in England, Morny Cannon, Wooton, Bullock, and that great favourite of the race fans, Steve Donoghue, are among the big names of that time.

Steve Donoghue

Steve Donoghue was born in Warrington, Lancashire, in 1884 and became the 'glamour boy' of the turf in the 1930s and 1940s. He was champion jockey and during a chequered career won the Epsom Derby four times, and came home twice the winner of the war-time substitute of the great classic at Newmarket. But, for people, his name

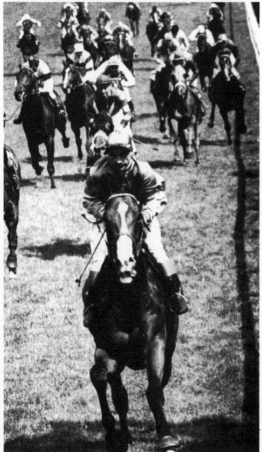

Above left *Since the revolution instigated by Todhunter Sloan fantastic results have been achieved. The principle of the 'monkey seat' was to balance the jockey's weight on the horse's withers allowing him to run freely and without impeding his natural galloping action.*

Above far left *The New Zealand-bred racehorse, Phar Lap. Considered by the Australians as one of the best-ever racers, he stunned America by his performances before dying in 1933 probably through accidental poisoning.*

Below far left *Donoghue, the best loved jockey in England since Fred Archer. He won every English Classic and was champion jockey for ten seasons.*

Below centre *Willie Shoemaker 'the midget millionaire' flails home Lucky Debonair in 1965.*

Below left *Sir Gordon Richards. Throughout his career one victory nearly eluded him – that of the Derby. In the year before his retirement and just after being knighted, he was at last successful on Pinza after 27 previous attempts.*

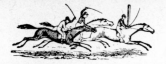

Opposite page *The finish of the 1922 Derby with Steve Donoghue in the lead on Captain Cuttle.*

Right *Although small and stocky, Gordon Richards was an immensely strong rider.*

Far right *Charlie Smirke takes the 1934 Epsom Derby after a five year suspension.*

Below *The Australian Scobie Breasley up on Santa Claus, the horse on which he finally took the winning honours in the Derby.*

Below right *George Moore pushing Royal Palace to victory.*

Bottom right *Eddie Arcaro on Nashua behind Swaps ridden by Willie Shoemaker in the 1955 Kentucky Derby.*

will always be linked with the great horse Brown Jack. These two had an uncanny relationship and together won the Queen Alexandra Stakes, a 'stayers' race at Ascot, no less than six times.

Tod Sloan's monkey seat had by now been generally adopted, streamlined and in some case improved upon. Two schools of thought were established and their differences became obvious and marked. One was to get the horse into his stride and going freely, then to let him make his own race trying to outrun the other horses. The other was to get the horse settled and relaxed,

running within his bounds of stamina then at the distance pole to nurse him up to the leaders keeping him always just ahead without unnecessary exertion.

Gordon Richards

Star jockeys of each school dominated world racing right up to the super-efficient 1960s and 1970s. One of these riders was Gordon Richards, a man born to be a jockey. Standing no more than 1·5m (4ft 11in) in his racing boots, this great jockey, 26 times champion of England, had the

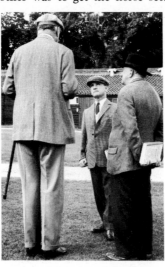

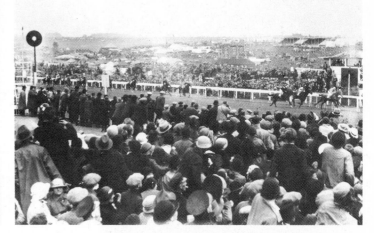

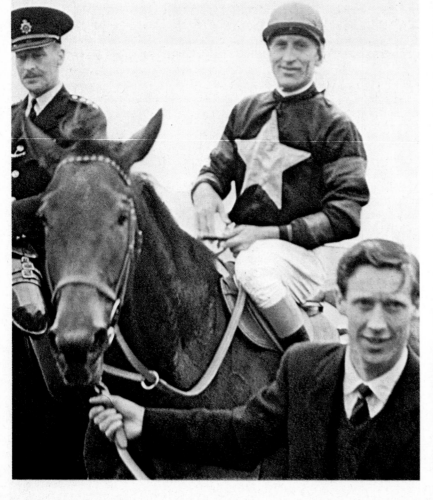

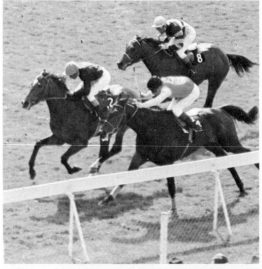

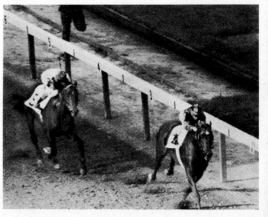

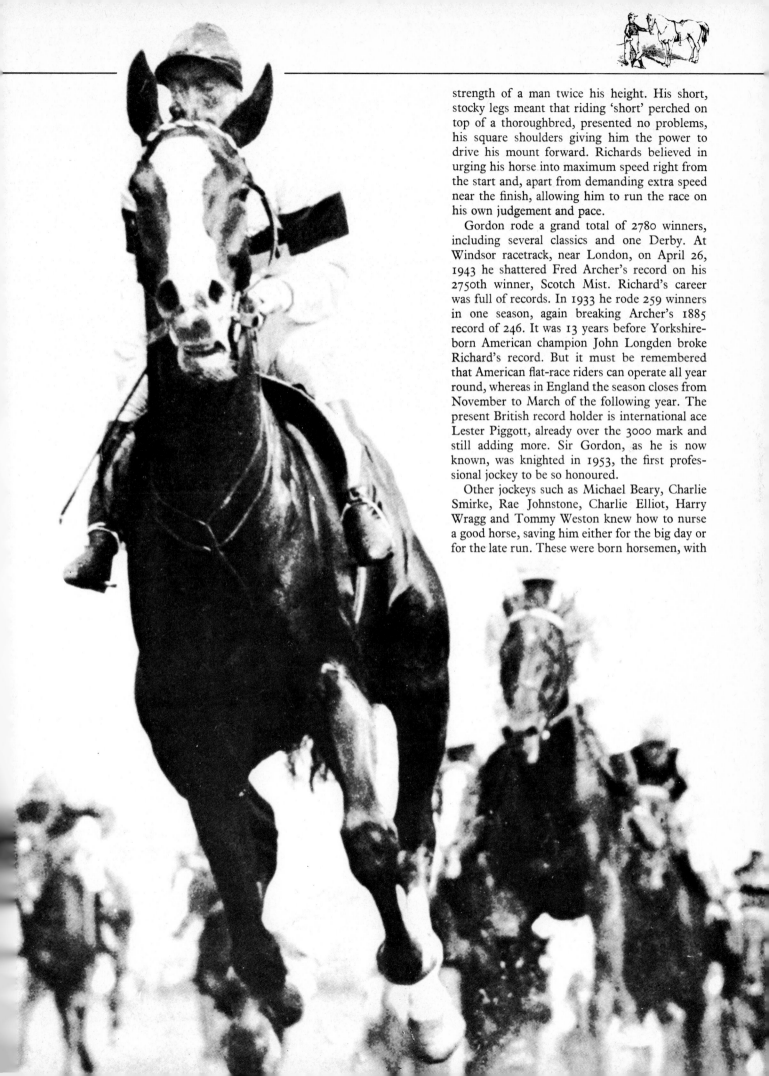

strength of a man twice his height. His short, stocky legs meant that riding 'short' perched on top of a thoroughbred, presented no problems, his square shoulders giving him the power to drive his mount forward. Richards believed in urging his horse into maximum speed right from the start and, apart from demanding extra speed near the finish, allowing him to run the race on his own judgement and pace.

Gordon rode a grand total of 2780 winners, including several classics and one Derby. At Windsor racetrack, near London, on April 26, 1943 he shattered Fred Archer's record on his 2750th winner, Scotch Mist. Richard's career was full of records. In 1933 he rode 259 winners in one season, again breaking Archer's 1885 record of 246. It was 13 years before Yorkshire-born American champion John Longden broke Richard's record. But it must be remembered that American flat-race riders can operate all year round, whereas in England the season closes from November to March of the following year. The present British record holder is international ace Lester Piggott, already over the 3000 mark and still adding more. Sir Gordon, as he is now known, was knighted in 1953, the first professional jockey to be so honoured.

Other jockeys such as Michael Beary, Charlie Smirke, Rae Johnstone, Charlie Elliot, Harry Wragg and Tommy Weston knew how to nurse a good horse, saving him either for the big day or for the late run. These were born horsemen, with

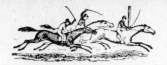

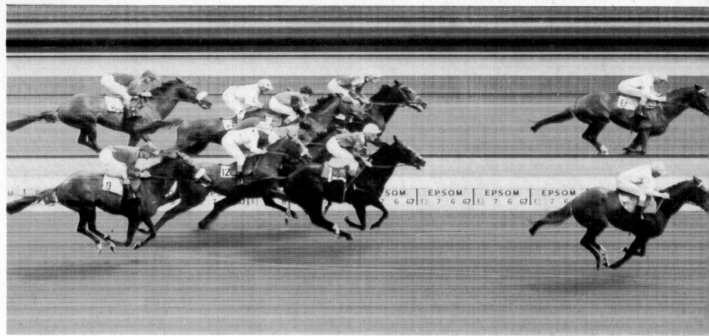

Above *How the photo-finish camera saw the finish of the 1967 Derby. Although today an accepted part of equipment on the race track, before the Second World War many race results were the subject of much controversy.*

Right *They're off! Few race courses allow this type of start today – most having starting gates to ensure a fair start for all competitors.*

Above right *Lester Piggott canters Sir Ivor gently down to the starting gate for the beginning of the Eclipse Stakes.*

Below far right *The popularity of racing is such that race courses can be found in all settings such as this seaside course at Brighton.*

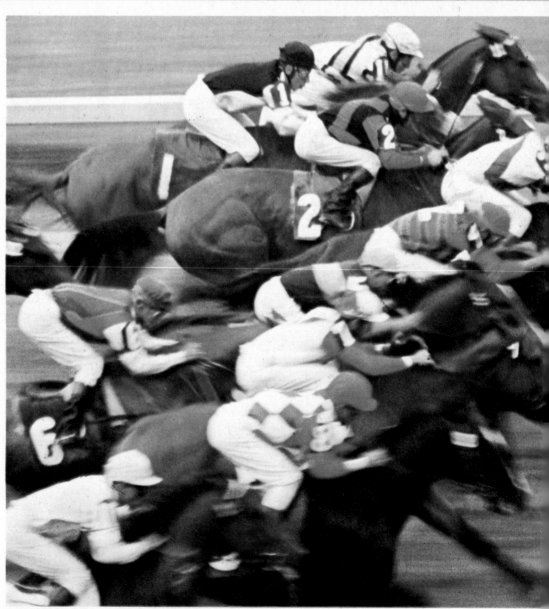

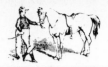

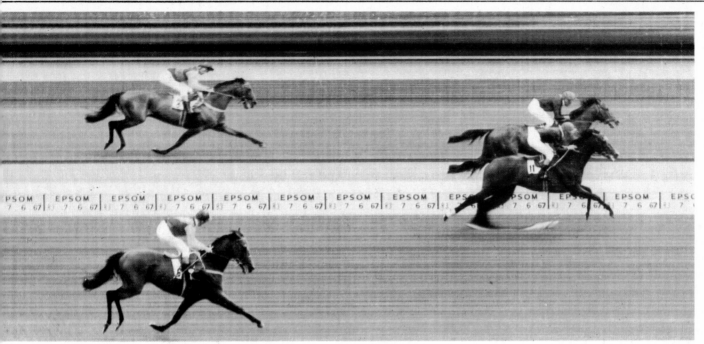

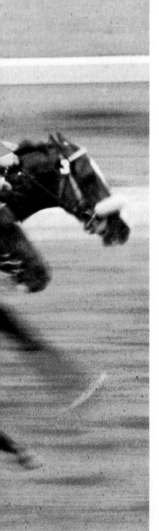

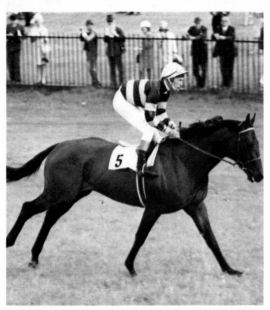

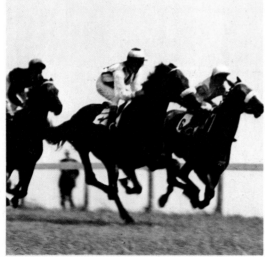

hands as gentle as a mother's and brains as sharp as any poker player. Like the early barbarian chieftains, these men could scream and shout with the best of them or sit it out quietly at the back, waiting for the right moment to pounce.

Acey Deucy Technique

In America Johnny Longden, Eddie 'Banana-nose' Arcaro, William Shoemaker, Bill Hartak and Braulio Baeza perfected the technique created by Sloan, and added one other refinement to the crouching seat. Although there are some American grass tracks, most of the race strips are dirt-tracks, and the layout, as against European courses, is sharp and circular. To be able to balance his mount all the way round, the American jockey rides with what is known as the 'Acey-Deucy' technique. This means that he has one stirrup-leather longer than the other. For example, on a right-handed track, his right leather would be slightly longer, enabling him to lean his weight to the right and encourage his horse to lean into the barrier. On a left-handed circuit the left leather would be slightly longer. Most American jockeys are naturally small and they sit tightly bunched to their horse's body, encouraging him to stretch out at the rushing ground before them. Because American training techniques are based on the stopwatch, their judgement of pace is as accurate as a speedometer.

In France, the native-born jockeys made their presence felt in the form of Roger Poincelet, crack jockey to the powerful Boussac stable, Jean Deforge, Georges Bridgland, Jacques Doyasbere, Georges Thiboeuf and the now brilliant Yves St Martin.

Australian Aces

In the years after World War II, the Australian jockey was the most sought after on the inter-

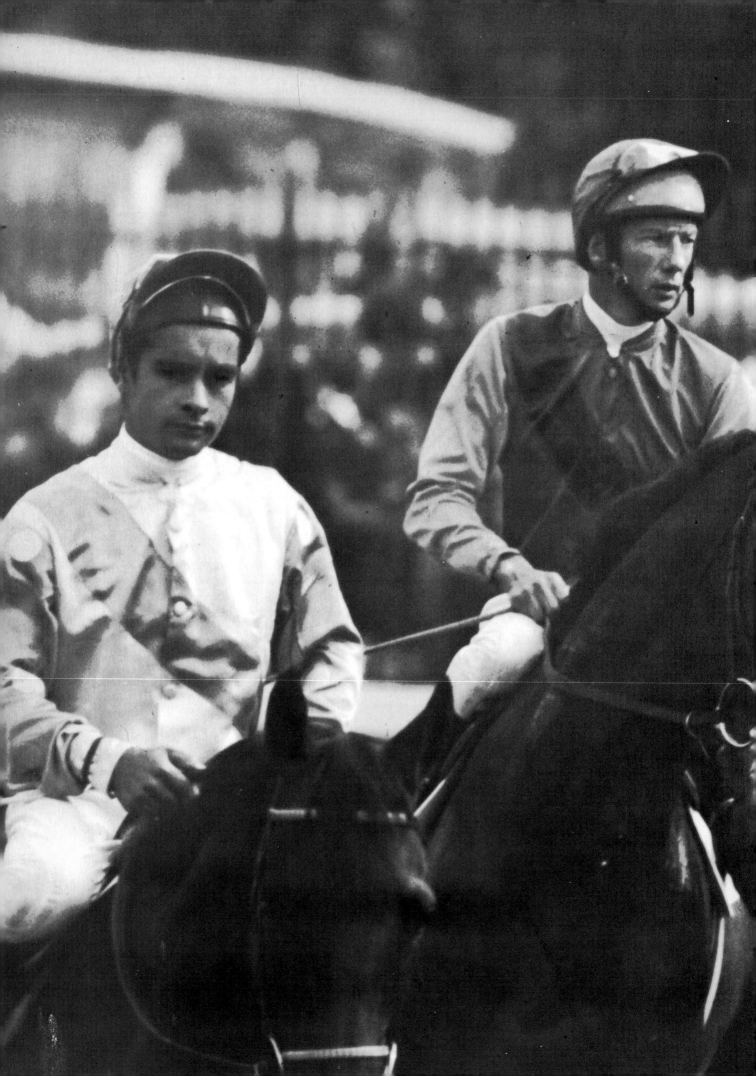

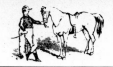

national circuit. This young nation in the racing sense produces jockeys capable of adapting quickly to the European or American systems. They are natural horsemen with superb hands. They can ride a waiting race, or go off in front, whichever is required. Like their American counterparts they are masters at judging pace to the stopwatch. Many Australian aces have ridden with great success in Europe. Notable are Edgar Britt, who rode in England, Rae Johnstone, who was based in France but was known as a 'Derby' specialist, Willy Cook, Garnie Bougoure, Scobie Breasley and George Moore. Breasley became a champion jockey in England and was a master of the waiting technique. He is now a successful trainer at Epsom, the home of the Derby.

George Moore was, perhaps, the finest jockey Australia has ever produced. Now a trainer in Hong Kong, he first hit the headlines in France under contract to the then all-conquering Marcel Boussac stable. But it was not until he signed to ride for England's number one trainer, Noel Murless, that he was able to show his real talent as a world-class horseman and jockey. A very fine horseman, George Moore had the special talent of getting even the most wayward thoroughbred to co-operate with him. He did not wave his whip and entered a starting box on a long loose rein, rubbing his mount's mane or neck. At the start he tried to get out with a clean balanced break and then let the horse settle and relax. But in the home straight he would appear from nowhere, taking his mount past the post with the minimum of effort. In one extremely successful year with the Murless stable in 1967, George won the 2000 Guineas on Royal Palace, the 1000 Guineas on Fleet, the Derby, once again on Royal Palace, and practically all the leading handicaps of that season.

Lester Piggott

The new style jockey with his private 'plane and complicated contracts has taken over. Lester Piggott, the 'enfant terrible' of the English tracks in his formative years, is generally accepted as the finest living jockey. Champion jockey of England, he has been the rider of classic winners all over the world, including six English Derbys, two 2000 Guineas, one 1000 Guineas, four winners of the Oaks, seven St Legers, the Derby winners of practically all the Continental countries including the Prix de L'Arc de Triomphe, and major wins in Ireland and the United States. This is the record of the greatest jockey of all time. Lester, with his individual flamboyant style, can ride four important races in four different countries in one working week.

Yves St Martin

In France, now one of the most important and powerful racing nations, Yves St Martin is the current leading flat-race jockey. St Martin is the only reinsman capable of matching Piggott at his own game, with his powerful rhythmic way of

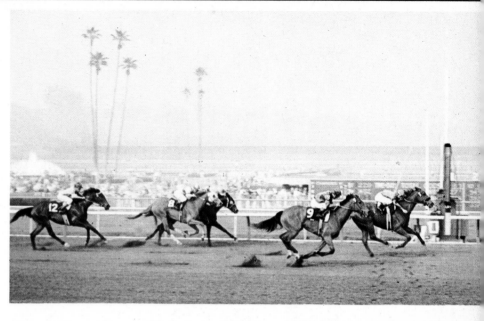

riding his horses flat out. Where Lester Piggott's style is full of many, idiosyncratic flourishes, St Martin's is pared down to essentials. He has proved himself beyond the courses of Longchamp and Chantilly, riding the winners of one 1000 Guineas and one Epsom Derby on the legendary Relko, and the Irish Oaks.

During the last 50 years thoroughbred breeding and racing has developed into a vast, international industry, with state-owned studs being established in England, Ireland, France, Italy, Russia and other countries. In America and the continental countries in particular, centralized racing has been brought to a fine art and tote-monopoly betting systems contribute a great deal of money to the community or the state.

The racecourses

The racecourse is the universe of peoples of all walks of life. It is a sanctuary for connoisseurs of the thoroughbred, a meeting place for gamblers, aristocracy, mannequins, journalists, industrialists, taxi-drivers and family men. There are restaurants, children's play-areas, closed circuit television and open areas to sit in the sun between races. Each country has its special tracks and big dates in the sporting calendar. In England it is Epsom for the Derby—a real fiesta day with gypsies, fun-fairs, and charabancs lining the rails of its famous long, sweeping home turn, Tattenham Corner. Or Ascot in Berkshire, where the Royal meeting is run every year and is the fashion show of the racing world. In France, Longchamp and Chantilly are the most popular tracks. Longchamp, sited right in the middle of Paris, is one of the most modern racetracks in Europe. Its vast grandstand dominates the home stretch. This is the stage for the Prix de L'Arc de Triomphe, now the richest race in the world. A few kilometres outside Paris is the more natural course, Chantilly. In the Prix du Jockey Club (the French Derby) the horses run down the back stretch past the majestic stable building of the

Above *American horses fight out the last few yards at Santa Anita on a dirt track typical of those in the United States.*

Opposite page *Two great rivals from modern racing world – Yves St Martin (left) and Lester Piggott before the start of the 1970 St Leger.*

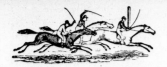

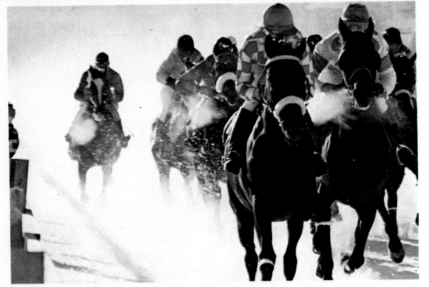

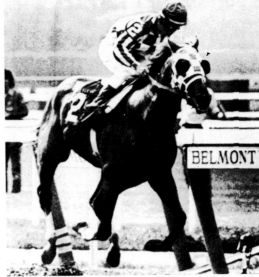

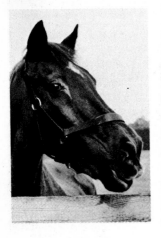

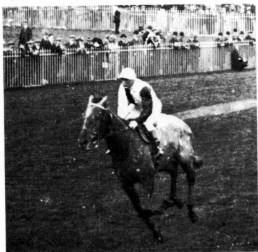

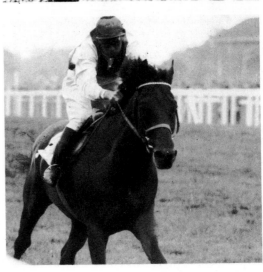

Above *Hyperion after a short but relatively successful racing career proved a prolific sire, eleven of his progeny winning the Classics.*

Top *In a flurry of snow horses at St Moritz race to an exciting finish.*

Above right *One of the great horses from the history of racing. The unbeaten Tetrarch winning the 1913 Champagne Stakes at Doncaster, as a two year old. He later became a leading branch of the Byerley Turk line.*

old Chateau, and then downhill to the final turn and the slightly raised, testing home straight.

The most famous track in America is in Aqueduct, Long Island. It is a fast circular course with its centre landscaped into ornamental lakes. On the days of any big race at Aqueduct or Belmont Park, the other New York track, the traffic going to the course is so dense that it takes four hours to cover 16km (10 miles). Hollywood Park, Los Angeles is the biggest of American racetracks. There, 1552 individual stalls have been built to accommodate the horses trained. Less spacious but still beautifully laid out are Laurel Park, Maryland, scene of the annual Washington International, Hileah, in Miami, and two of the oldest tracks in the United States, Pimlico, Baltimore and Saratoga in the State of New York. In Kentucky, the horse breeding state of America, can be found the Keeneland racecourse, with one of the most famous bloodstock sales rings attracting buyers from all parts of the world prepared to pay the highest prices for a potential winner. But the real history of modern racing, like its romantic grass-roots era, is not just about human stars or fine racecourses, but the vital commodity of the sport—legendary horses

Hyperion

Hyperion, a small chestnut, is one horse whose influence on thoroughbred breeding throughout the world has yet to be surpassed. Standing only slightly over 15 hands he was a horse of perfect conformation and action. He won the 1933 Epsom Derby in record time and went on to take the St Leger at Doncaster in the same year, beating a good field with nonchalant ease. He was the leading sire of winners in England on six occasions and his son Aureole, owned and raced by Queen Elizabeth II, was also a leading classic sire of his generation. Two more of his sons, Heliopolis and Alibhai, brought their father's bloodline into the American racehorse.

Man O'War

Man O'War, or Big Red as American race fans called him, was a great crowd-puller. Born in 1917 and bought for $5000 (£2092), Big Red ran in 21 races and was only beaten on one occasion, after he had started badly. Over a career spanning 30 years he earned his owner more than one million dollars (£418,000) from prize money, stud fees and the sales of his foals. He was the father of the gallant little Battleship that came to

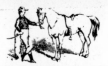

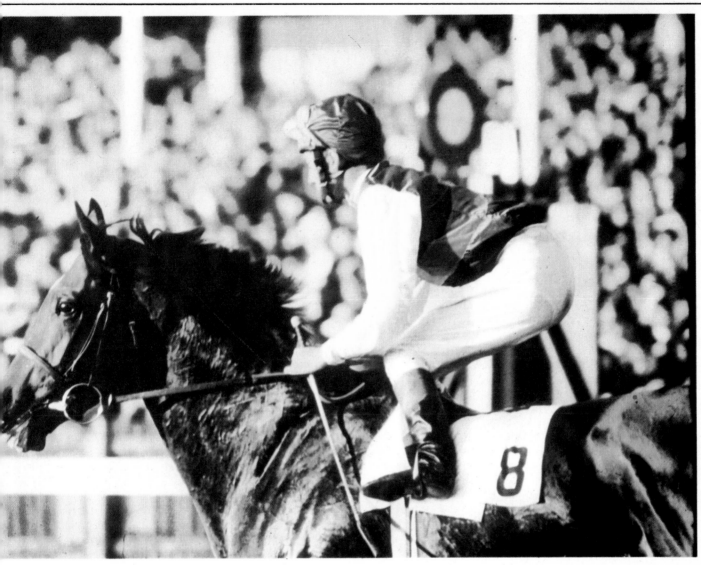

England in 1938 and won the Grand National. In the years after his retirement from the track he received over one and a half million visitors, finally dying of a heart attack in 1947.

Buckpasser

Buckpasser was another of America's equine 'millionaires' winning $1,462,014 (£620,089) in prize money from 21 races out of 31 starts. American horses have dominated the post-war racing scene, with such horses as Native Dancer, who won 21 out of 22 races, his only defeat being in the Kentucky Derby, sold as a stallion for well over one million dollars, Secretariat and Riva Bridge, both classic winners and now standing at stud.

In England and Ireland, each season produces an outstanding horse, such as the American-bred Sir Ivor, winner of the 2000 Guineas and the Epsom Derby in 1968. Mill Reef and Brigadier Gerard, two great rivals, were unlucky to be born at the same time and produced some of the greatest races of recent years. Brigadier Gerard won the 2000 Guineas in 1971 and Mill Reef went on to take the Derby and run out one of the easiest winners in the tough Prix de L'Arc de Triomphe. Although Mill Reef met with a training accident which put an end to his racing career, his life was saved, thanks to the immense advances in veterinary science, and he now stands at stud, as does his old rival Brigadier Gerard.

Italy's greatest racehorse has undoubtedly been Ribot who only ran sixteen times but was never beaten. He won all the Italian classics and the Prix de L'Arc de Triomphe in 1955 and 1956. He came to England and thrilled fans with a six-length victory in the valuable King George VI and Queen Elizabeth Stakes at Ascot. He stood at stud in his native country and then in America, where he bred the American classic horses, Tom Rolfe, Dapper Dan and Arts and Letters.

There are many other horses whose careers would fill volumes. Sea Bird, Nijinsky, Gladiateur and The Tetrarch are some names still remembered. These are the real stars of racing and each and every one of them is in some way related. The blue blood that runs through their veins came from the same source: the three Arabian stallions imported after the reign of Charles II.

Above *The famous partnership of Lester Piggott and Nijinsky. Capable of the most spectacular wins at times, Nijinsky took the English Triple Crown in 1970, the first horse to do so for 35 years.*

Above far left *Secretariat, the most outstanding of recent race horses crosses the line to take the American Triple Crown, the first horse to do so for 25 years.*

Below far left *Bred from Italian stock Ribot confounded all predictions for his future, never losing a race, his triumphs including 2 Prix de l'Arc de Triomphe and the King George VI and Queen Elizabeth Stakes.*

Showjumping -
unnatural & exacting -
the youngest of equestrian sports

The origins of show-jumping, the most exacting of equestrian sports, are obscure. Horse shows can be traced back to the latter part of the 18th century but these were mainly country agricultural shows. The horse events on the programmes were orientated more to the bloodstock angle of show horses than to jumping competitions.

The origins of show-jumping

From the very beginning, the art of show-jumping has always been to get over, if possible without touching, a series of man-made obstacles. Show-jumping is unique as an equestrian sport in that the horse is required to jump a series of obstacles within the confines of a man-made ring and in cold blood. In dressage the natural airs and graces of the horse are displayed. Racing, both flat and steeplechasing, is based on the animal's instinctive spirit of competition within the herd. The same is true of hunting, the oldest equestrian sport where man and horse are in their natural environment. In show-jumping, there are none of these natural stimulants. There is no herd from which to draw security. It is horse and rider out in a ring on their own.

The grass-roots of the sport seem to be divided between the soldier-riders of the great military schools, who enjoyed a sport then known as the High-Jump, and the dealers, with their jumping events on the village green. It seems more likely that it was the dealers who, to prove how good their horses were and to sell them for good prices, first competed in true show-jumping competitions. In contrast, the military rider had an endless string of army horses to call upon and competition for him was more a question of showing how good he was as a horseman rather than to demonstrate the brilliance of the horse. He did not have to attract the eyes of a potential buyer and jumping horses over fences became an absorbing pastime.

On the Continent the military rider completely dominated equestrian sport outside racing. And he took the idea of show-jumping more seriously than did his English equivalent. More thought was given to the construction of fences and courses. The 'show' aspect of the sport was the attraction for the continental rider. Because of his traditions and natural understanding of dressage, which overawed the English rider, he saw show-jumping as a test as well as a competition. The courses were therefore laid out with a mixture of natural and unnatural fences and the siting or distances between each was carefully worked out to test the horse's obedience as well as his jumping ability.

In the early 1900s, before the World War I, the courses and system of judging in England were very different from their modern equivalents. The competitions were basically of two types. The first consisted of a small, short course of obstacles. The second was what was then known as the Touch-and-out, Knock-and-out, Single-bar or more simply and, perhaps more accurately, the High-jump. This was simply one fence, usually a single bar. The fence started off quite low, then with each round it was raised a notch at a time. Any competitor knocking the bar down could not go into the next round. Sometimes it would go as high as 1·8m (6ft). If the winning horse was owned by a dealer he would be promptly surrounded by prospective buyers.

The obstacle courses were very simple, consisting of some four to six fences, not given a great deal of technical thought, dotted around the ring. These were not as demanding as continental fences. The rider did not have to make any changes of rein. The fences, which were mainly uprights, would be sited in a uniform pattern, three along one side, three (or sometimes two and two) along the other side. And on very rare occassions a spread or water jump was placed in the middle. So that, nine times out of ten, the rider always used his right rein.

In those amateur days show-jumping had no strong governing body and although most of the village-green shows used the same rules, they were by no means constant. If the horse hit the pole with his front legs he collected two faults. If he hit a fence with the hind-legs he collected four faults. But there was little chance of getting away with tapping a pole—for on each was placed a thin slat of wood and if this was dislodged the competitor was faulted as if he had knocked down the bar. In many areas this system of scoring was reversed. Four faults were given for a hit with front legs and two faults for a hit with the hind-legs. The rule on refusals or taking the wrong course was more or less the same as today. A third refusal at a particular fence meant elimination. The time element was not considered in competition jumping at that time.

The natural and physical schools

The horse is not a natural jumper like other members of the animal kingdom. The 'natural school' of riding believes that the horse can be

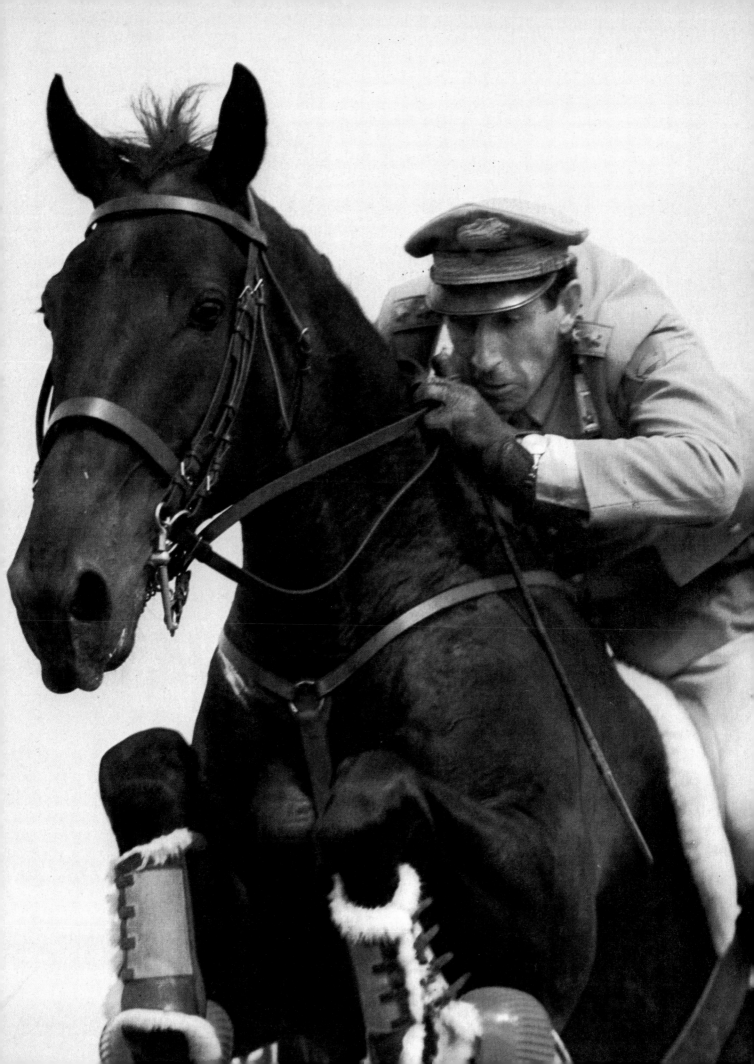

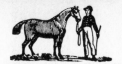

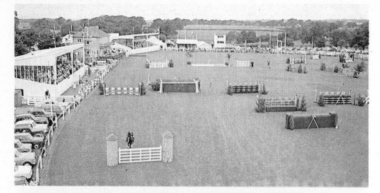

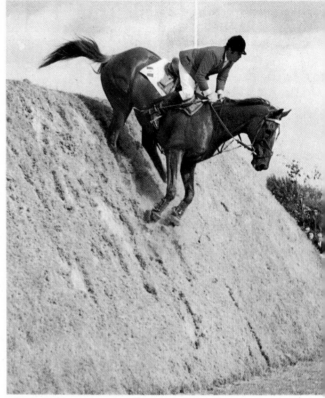

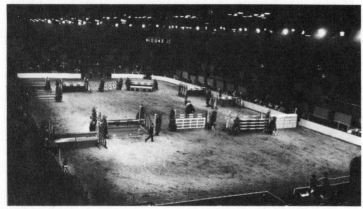

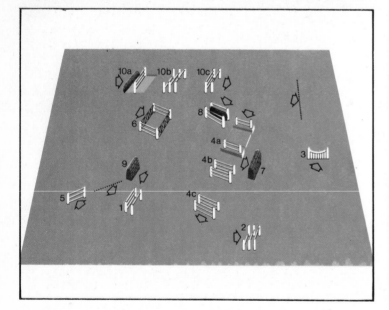

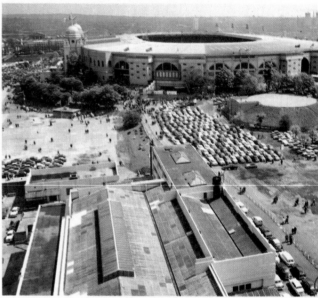

educated to think for himself, and, with the minimum interference from the rider, to jump his fences fluently. For this a quality horse is needed, and a rider with patience, time and a lot of experience of getting horses fit and supple. The results are good to watch, and consistent.

The 'physical school' of riding believes that the horse can be trained to obey his rider completely and that by putting the animal in more complicated gear the rider can shorten or lengthen the stride whenever he thinks it desirable. A horse of lesser quality can be used and the training is quicker. The end-product is exciting to watch, but the results are inconsistent.

The two systems have a common, basic founda-

tion. This is to ask, or force, a horse to jump several artificial obstacles, an unnatural task for the horse. Whether the rider trains the horse through the use of equipment and discipline or whether he allows the horse to teach itself, the end-product, although different to the eye, is the same package: the horse jumps from the rhythm of his stride and the use of his body. Some people call it 'spring', but the horse is not a 'springing' type of creature. The idea is to arrive at the obstacle in such a cadence as to unleash the power of the stride at a balanced moment, the point of take-off. Muscle power is what makes the horse jump. In modern jumping, the fences are laid out in such a manner that (a) they must

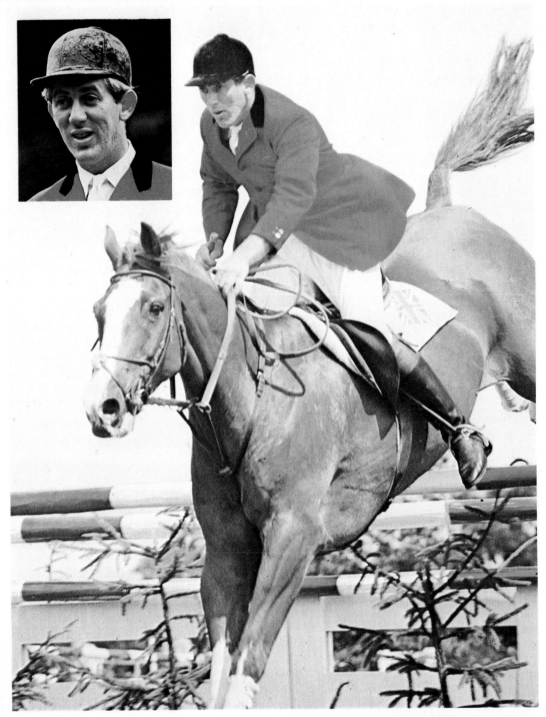

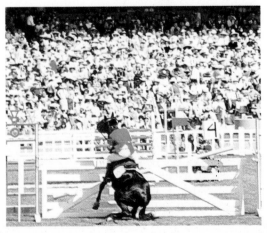

Left *One of the finest natural horsemen in the world, ex-World Champion David Broome on Mr Softee the horse with which he won two Men's European Championships. But it was on the boisterous Beethoven that he took the World Championship.*

Below *The horse not only faces the jump but in a championship arena, the crowded backdrop can also provide a problem to the unsettled horse.*

Opposite page top right and left *Two views of Britain's Hickstead arena. A course should produce the top horse and rider combination and provide entertaining sport for the spectators.*

Opposite page centre left and bottom right *Venue of many international equestrian events – the Wembley Stadium.*

Opposite page left *The course for a CHIO grand prix event; approx. 450 metres long, the rider is limited to 76 seconds to get round.*

be jumped and not knocked down, (b) they must be approached correctly, the distances being calculated to test horse's and rider's technique and training, and (c) the jumps cannot be treated individually but must be regarded as a whole. One system is not better than the other in terms of results. Most modern teams take the best points and with great success use a combination of both systems.

The improved courses

Between 1918 and the early 1930s the show-jumping courses improved. They became slightly longer and a water jump was often included. But they were still mainly composed of upright or

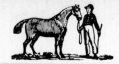

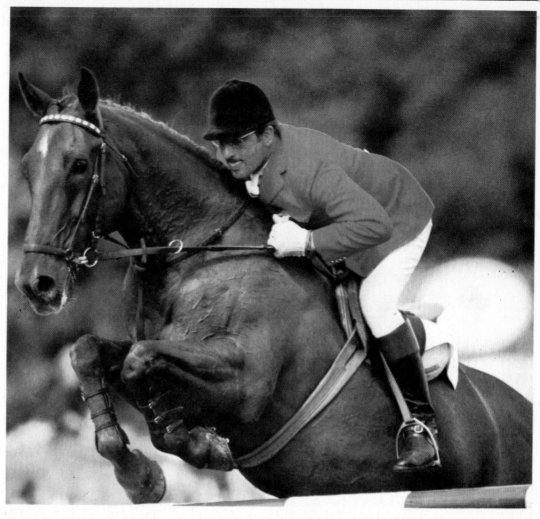

Right *In a long showjumping career, Hans Gunter Winkler, has won probably more prizes than any other leading show jumper. In the Munich Olympic Games he continued his run of successes by riding Torphy in the winning team.*

Opposite page *Pierre d'Oriola on Nagir. One of the first civilians to break into the predominately military French teams he has since taken two individual Gold medals at the Olympic Games and took the Men's World Championships in Buenos Aires in 1966.*

'straight' fences. Because of this, they tended to encourage the horseman who trained his horses to jump only one type of fence. As competition began to develop, a style of show-jump riding known as 'stop and start' evolved. In this style, the rider restrained his horse between each fence, only letting him go when asking him to jump. If a course consisted of upright fences only, and the top bars of those fences had light slats on them the rider was forced to think about precision rather than technique. So that the non-thorough-bred or lesser-quality horse was favoured. This type of horse, being less sensitive, would not become over-excited by the stopping and start-ing. In contrast, the thoroughbred horse, being more spirited, would become over-excited, termed 'hot-up' in show-jumping jargon, when ridden in this manner.

To understand this further, it is necessary to analyze how the show-jumping rider sees a course. The most important phase of any form of jumping is the approach to the fence and this is particularly so in show-jumping, where a high degree of accuracy is the object of the game. The horse measures a fence from the bottom up, looks for his point of take-off and then jumps. The rider must also be capable of judging this point of take-off so that he can go with the horse without being a hindrance to him. Because of

this show-jumping riders work on the technique of what is called 'seeing the stride'. This means that the rider prepares his horse, on coming into his fence, to arrive at a certain point that will give him a powerful take-off and every chance of clearing the obstacle.

The rider intends coming to the fence with his horse straight and balanced, at the same time restricting his mount with his hands, with his seat and his legs, encouraging the horse to be active particularly with his hind-legs. The horse is driven from behind—so that the more active and energy-producing the hindquarters are, the more power the horse will release when lifting himself into the air. When the rider feels he is approaching the fence correctly, and that his horse is active and balanced, he then pushes the horse into the fence. At the point of take-off he releases the horse's head so that the animal can use his body to go into the air and over the fence.

The upright fences of the 1930s required all the same timing, stride and technique, producing a sameness in the standard of equitation and a boring repetitiveness for the spectator. For up-right fences, it is height of jump for which the rider aims. So that he must hold up his horse for much longer to achieve maximum energy in the hindquarters releasing extra power to produce the height required. Because the rider waits until

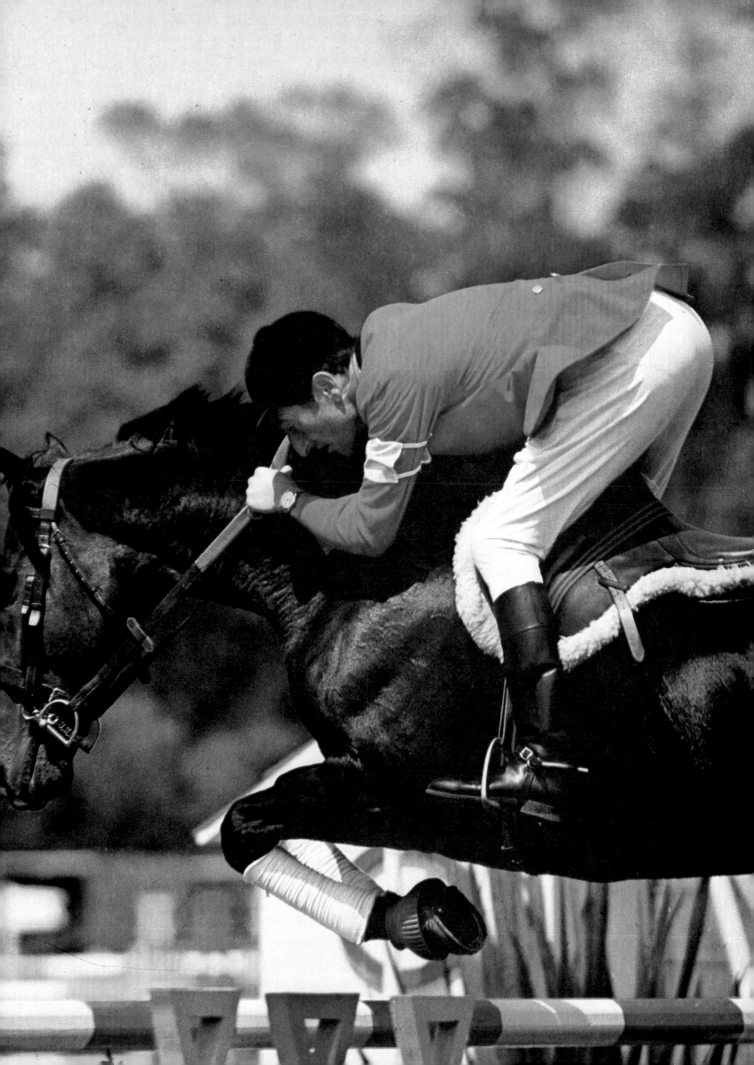

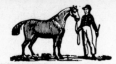

Right *Rome's beautiful Piazza di Siena, scene of the Italian Prix des Nations. The Prix des Nations is a team event for the Presidents Cup, instigated in 1965, on which is based the world team championship.*

Below *Dawn Palethorpe had a short but successful career in show jumping. Seen here riding Earlsrathe Rambler, on which she took the 1954 Ladies National title, she also represented Britain on a number of occasions before retiring to due to family commitments.*

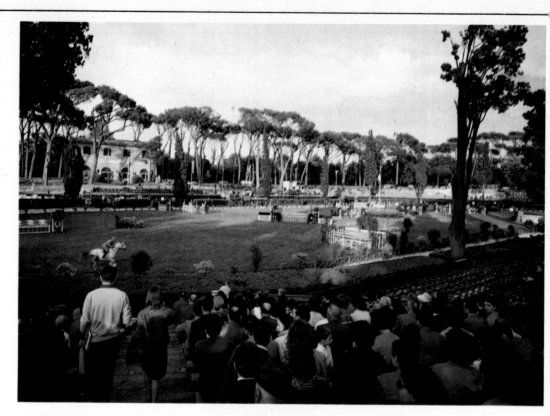

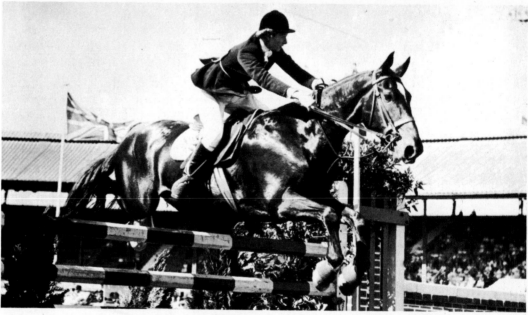

he is much closer to the fence before 'pushing' the horse on and up, the space between each fence is used for restricting the horse's forward momentum while he is at the same time asked to create activity and energy.

In modern show-jumping, on the other hand, there is a greater variety of fences, uprights, spreads, water, banks, dykes and parallels, so that the rider and the horse must be better trained and more scientific in their technique. To jump a spread, for example, the horse will need to approach faster and with a longer stride in order to be able to reach for the length. This may then be followed by an upright so the horse must be sufficiently supple and obedient to come back to the shorter stride on the approach to obtain the height.

The system of using straight upright fences was the recognized style of jumping in pre-war Britain and Ireland. It was a monotonous system but a successful one. And as most of the competitors were dealers or dealer's sons, dedicated to winning and selling, it tended to last and be copied by young riders. On the continent, where the competitors were mainly military personnel looking for prestige wins, the approach to the techniques of show-jumping was more scientific. Testing by distances was their idea of show-jumping, and for this they used a better-quality horse. With the exchange of ideas between riders

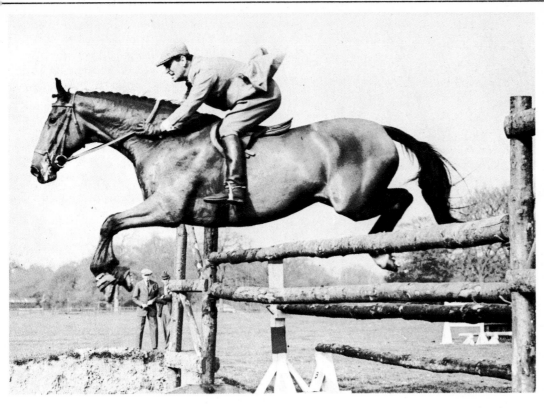

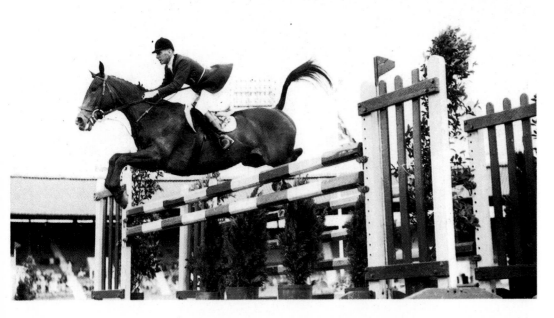

on national teams, the continental idea began to spread, but the effects of this evolution on show-jumping were not to be seen until after World War II.

The course with its fences is the basic setting of the sport. But it was not until the post-war years that the occupation of course-builder became recognized as an essential part of the game. Prior to that time it was very much an ad-lib affair. Whoever had the time or the materials would agree to erect some jumps and there was little thought or planning involved. But with the upsurge of interest in horses which occurred just after the war it was soon realized that people would come to see a horse show if it

was entertaining. To encourage the public the courses changed and variety in the type of fence evolved. Spread fences came into use, as did double and treble combination fences and better ground-lines and wings, which changed the face of show-jumping techniques. The better-trained horse and the more scientific rider came into his own.

In the 1950s the courses began to be designed as well as constructed. Lieutenant-Colonel Jack Talbot-Ponsonby, one of the all-time greats as a rider, brought the science of course building to England. His courses were big and complicated but they only posed problems for the talented horse and rider, never riddles. The fluent jumper

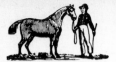

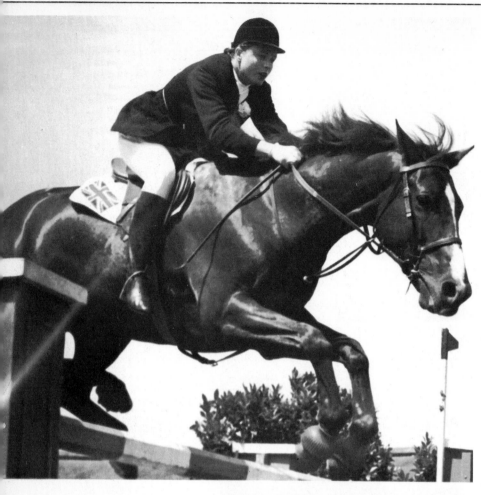

took over from where the precision rider had left off. The rules were standardized by the now-strong British Show Jumping Association, which is affiliated to the Federation Equestre Internationale, the world-governing body of equestrian sports.

Simplicity was the keynote to the new rules. For knocking down a fence, four faults were given; for a refusal, three faults; a second refusal, six faults and a third refusal at the same fence, elimination. For taking the wrong course, elimination. The time element was introduced. A maximum time was allowed for each competition so that if the horse and rider fell they were not directly penalized but they incurred time faults. Speed competitions and timed jump-offs provided spectators with plenty of excitement as horses and riders tried to beat the clock on the run for the line.

The aim of the course builder is to construct a series of fences that will encourage flowing movement, bold jumping and natural, free riding. This he can do in several ways, depending on the time and material at his disposal. A great deal also depends on the knowledge the course builder has of the horse and equitation. An ex-show-jumping rider, such as Jack Talbot-Ponsonby or Hans Heinrich Brinkmann of Germany, give proof to this. Both were Olympic riders and both have become legends as course builders. Riders like their courses and horses jump them well. As they have practical experience of what it is like to jump in top-class competition their sympathy for the horse and their refusal to trap him with a dangerous fence makes any track built by them the finest that can be seen.

It is not absolutely essential that a course builder should be an ex-show-jumping rider. The technique of constructing a course can be taught to anybody who has the slightest idea of how to read a plan and use a tape-measure and yard-stick. In the lower grades of competition this is really all that is required of a course builder. But at international standards it is very rare indeed for someone who is not fully conversant with the art of riding competition horses to be capable of building a course that really tests the top-class performer and entertains the spectators at the same time.

The ideal show-jumping course should be planned to suit the standard and ability of the entries and should be a good test of jumping and horsemanship. The fences must be wide enough to encourage a good approach. A width of about 4·5m (15ft) is the most suitable. The wings of the jump must be obvious to the eye, by their height, colour or material. Trees, shrubs or flowers make perfect dressings for the wings. This will help the horse and rider to focus on the line of the fence. Consecutive fences should be blended as closely as possible, through the use of similar colours. If, for example, there is a line of four fences, or a combination of three fences, the horse's eye will be attracted down the line. If the

Above *Pat Smythe a leading rider in 1950s and 1960s on Mr Pollard. It was this horse that enabled her to win the Queen Elizabeth Cup in 1958.*

Right *But it was on Flanagan that she achieved most success becoming the first woman rider to compete in the Olympic Games and bringing back a bronze medal from Stockholm in 1956.*

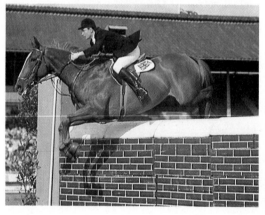

Below right *The famous combination in the early 1960s Piero D'Inzeo and the Rock, the great Irish-bred horse.*

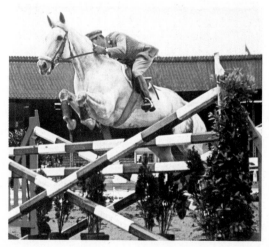

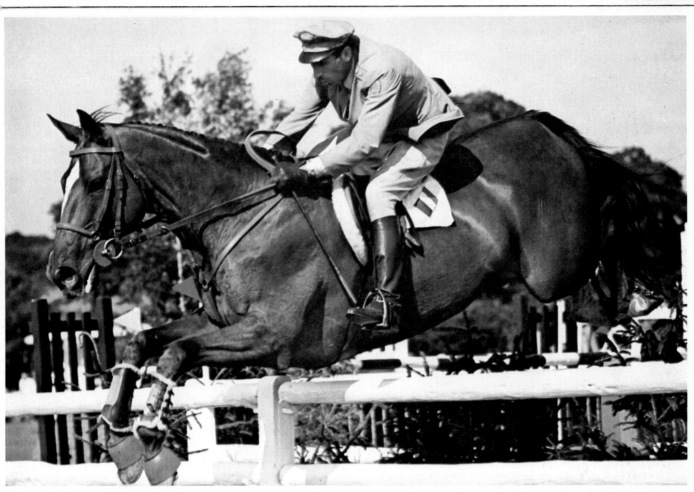

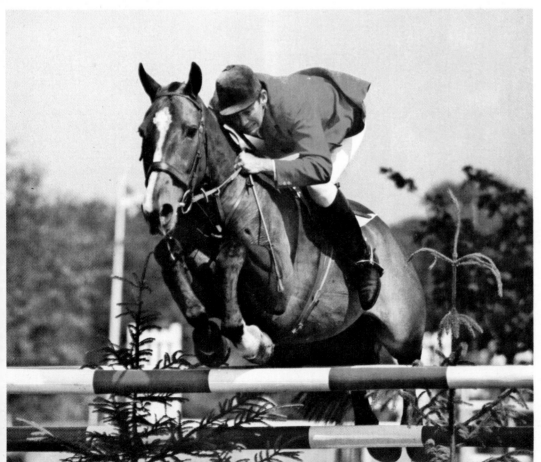

Above *Raimondo d'Inzeo on his 1968 World Championships mount, Bowjack.*

Left *Alan Oliver and Sweep III. Starting his career with an almost acrobatic style, he has now achieved considerable success with the more conventional approach of sitting tight.*

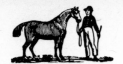

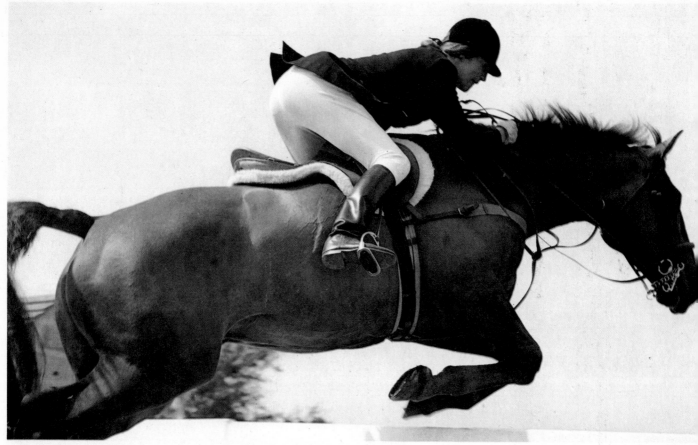

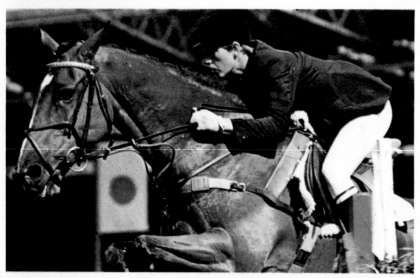

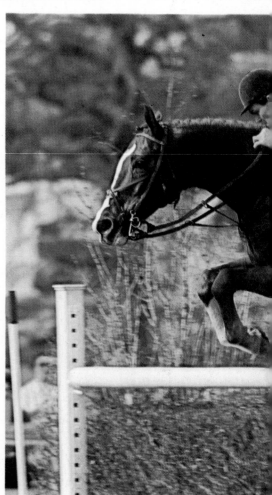

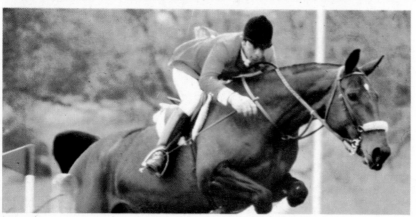

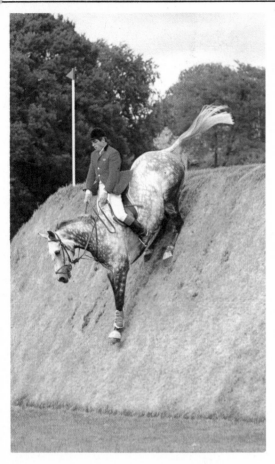

first fence is of red and white poles, and the second is a big rustic-coloured wall or oxer, the horse's eye will tend to look to the second fence as it will look startling. In doing so he will not concentrate on the first fence of the line but the second.

The solidness of fences can make them look easier to the horse. This may sound a contradiction in terms, but it is a fact that horses do not like flimsy fences. As their eyes are set on the sides of their heads they sight their fences from a distance, and if the fence is too flimsy or can be seen through too easily, the horse finds difficulty in measuring it. With the intelligent jumper this will cause worry, his concentration will be impaired and the performance will be poor.

The ground-lines of the fences must be well defined to encourage the horse to take the measure of his fence and then come in and jump it with confidence. Only courses designed for the really top-class performers can risk leaving out ground-lines. In America, for example, single bar and the six bar competitions are very popular. But the single bar is backed with a cross pole running diagonally across the frontage of the fence, and the six-bar type of fence has bars of the same colour. The fences are nearly always laid out in a direct and related line so that even at this advanced form of jumping no unfair difficulties are encountered by the horse or rider.

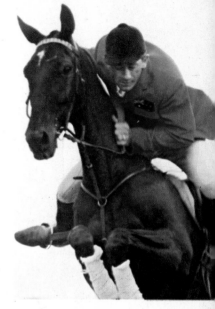

Above *The Australian Kevin Bacon on Chichester. Showjumpers come from many stocks, Chichester himself coming from a long line of racing and cattle ponies.*

Above left *Alwin Schockemohle coming down the bank at Hickstead.*

Above far left *Anneli Drummond Hay makes a perfect jump.*

Below left *Ted Edgar about to descend the Bank at Hickstead on his ex-rodeo horse Uncle Max.*

Below centre *The ever-popular Harvey Smith on O'Malley. In 1972 he became the first British rider to turn professional and went into partnership with Trevor Banks.*

Centre far left *Alison Dawes on Mr Banbury.*

Below far left *The Brazilian Nelson Pessoa won so many European events that the sport was forced to set up residential qualifications in non-international events.*

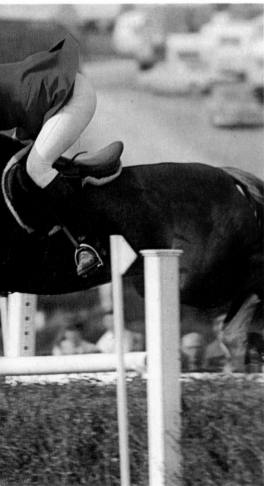

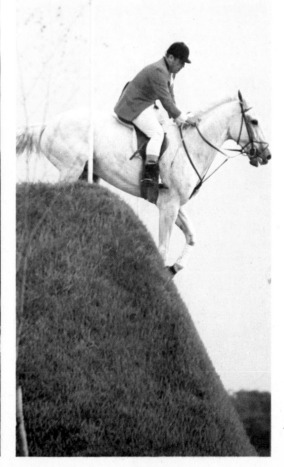

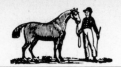

The intelligent course builder constructs and sites his first three or four fences so that they warm-up the horse and rider for the more compilcated tests to come. It is unfair to make the first few fences too stiff or tricky. It also tends to spoil the competition for the spectators. There is no more beautiful sight than a good horse jumping big, attractive fences with smoothness and grace. Equally, there is no more unpleasant sight than a good horse crashing into fences or falling.

Combinations, which can be two obstacles or three, are the most difficult to design well and to jump well. The distances between each part must be such that the horse can achieve an even jumping stride at each part. This can be done by making the first part solid and of an inviting construction. If the rider rides his first fence correctly, he will almost certainly have enough open space and confidence of approach to jump the other parts so that he finishes the combination ready and balanced for the remainder of the course.

The most important part the course builder can play in contributing to the test and spectacle of the sport is the ingredient of variety. Although the basic principles of show-jumping construction are based on two staples—the upright and the spread—there is tremendous scope for the imaginative builder. By alternating different types of fences, such as a treble or double combination, a parallel, a simple upright, a staircase, a pyramid, banks, water and walls, and placing them in order of difficulty around the arena, the builder can make the competition more interesting and exciting. The main thing he must avoid is overdressing his fences thereby blocking the view of the public. The spectator comes to see jumping and the course builder must arrange it so that they can do just that.

Early shows

Since its inception show-jumping, like other equestrian sports, has produced its quota of legendary horses and colourful and skilled riders. Its history is packed with incident, variety and a competitiveness which can be equal to that of flat-racing or steeplechasing. The first international show took place in Turin, Italy, in 1901. This was a mainly military affair with Italian officers riding against German officers, and was not really the beginning of the modern international circuit. The Royal Dublin Society had been founded in 1731 but it was not until 1868 that jumping became part of its programme in the form of leaping contests orientated to displaying a horse's potential for the hunting field. There were two contests, with only one fence in each. The high leap consisted of three bars that could be raised, and the wide leap was performed over wattle placed parallel to each other. The rules were rather vague and quite simply said, 'The obstacles are to be cleared to the satisfaction of the judges.' One can imagine the arguments that must have filled the bars after these contests

were decided. The prize money was £5 ($13) and £2 ($5) for each event.

The term leaping contest was dropped for jumping competitions in 1891, and in 1894 jumping became part of the spring show in Dublin. The rules were reorganized and judges were placed at each obstacle to award marks. Throughout this period ladies were not allowed to compete, but in 1919 a competition was introduced, which was restricted solely to lady riders. Then 1926 saw the dawning of the great international atmosphere that is now unique to the Dublin Show. Colonel Ziegler, responsible for buying horses on behalf of the Swiss Government, suggested that a competition should be held between the Swiss and the Irish Army riders. It was an immediate success, and international jumping has been part of Dublin, with its attractive ring and permanent obstacles, ever since. From 1881 the show has been at its present site at Balls Bridge, and over £500,000 has been spent on improving the facilities of the near 20-ha (50-acre) site.

The year of 1883 saw the birth of the great American international show, at Madison Square Garden, New York. One of the oldest indoor shows in the world, it started as a national show only but in 1909 Alfred Vanderbilt, the president of the show, invited overseas competitors to compete. Madison Square Garden is now one of the most important international venues on the North American circuit, with the Royal Winter Fair in Toronto, which was founded in 1925.

In the early 1900s, at a dinner at the Badminton Club in London, an idea of establishing an indoor international show in the British capital was voiced. From this after-dinner conversation came the Royal International Horse Show, staged at Olympia, London, in 1907. The first president of the show was the fifth Earl of Lonsdale and his committee comprised 10 Dukes, 9 Marquises, 36 Earls, 14 Viscounts and 78 Lords. But it was not until the late 1940s that things really started in English show-jumping. The late Tony Collings, a riding instructor, came up with the idea of a Horse of the Year Show, at the Harringay indoor arena in London. The aim of the show was to find the leading horse and pony, in all sections of equestrian sport, with the emphasis tending to be on the jumpers. The man who turned the idea into reality was an ex-international rider and the recognized father of modern show-jumping in Britain, Sir Michael Ansell. He had planned the new style that show-jumping was to take while a prisoner-of-war in World War II. The Horse of the Year Show is now held annually at Wembley, London.

Foxhunter and Nizefela

The public soon made stars of the leading riders and equine personalities, such as Harry Llewellyn and the great Foxhunter. Foaled in 1940, this strong bay gelding, half thoroughbred half Clydesdale, represented Great Britain 35 times and had

Above right *Even some of the best riders make mistakes. Here Ballywillwill swerves to run out from the fence and loses his rider, David Broome.*

Below right *Austrian Hugo Simon on his beautiful grey Hanoverian-bred Lavendal.*

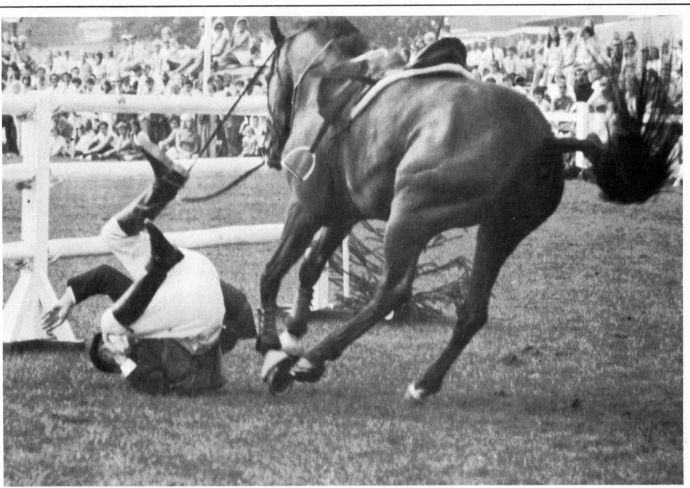

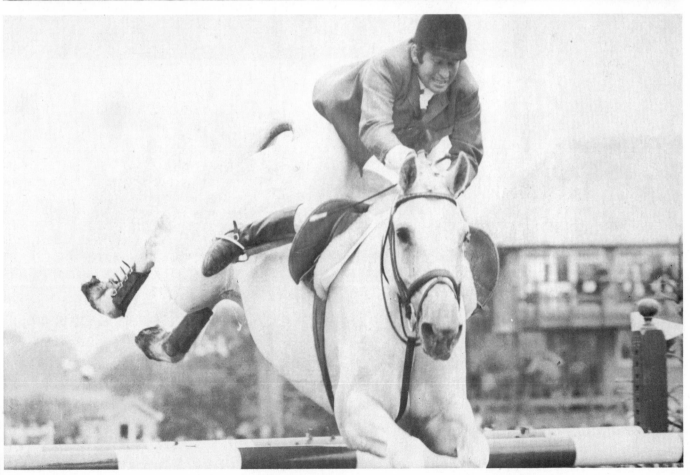

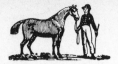

Right *Kathy Kusner the first non-European to win the Women's European title in 1967. She also became the first woman to hold a jockey's licence in the United States.*

Below right *One of the new string of American riders who excelled in Europe in 1974. Rodney Jenkins on Number One Spy.*

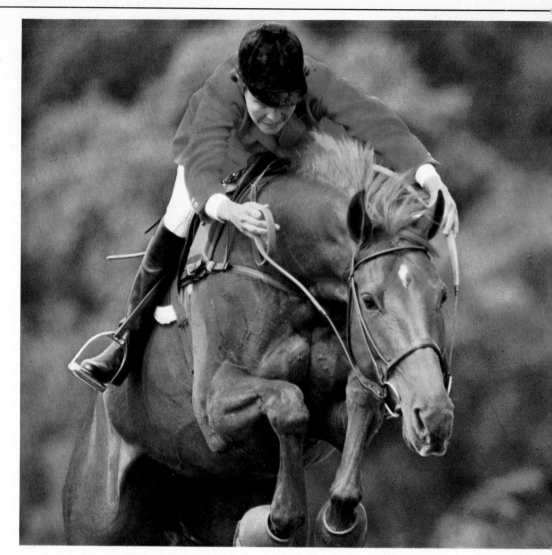

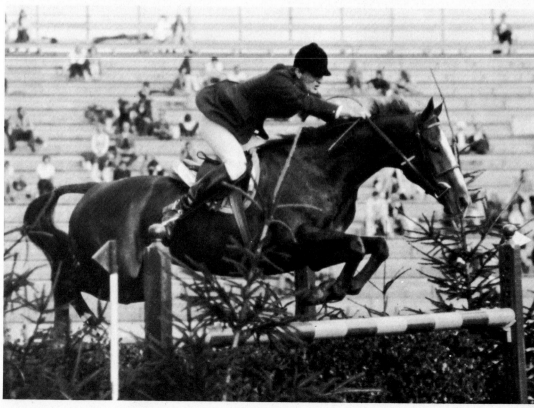

78 international wins to his credit. He won the King George V Cup three times, one of the most coveted prizes in show-jumping. Colonel Llewellyn semi-retired his famous partner in 1953 and three years later made their final farewell to the competition arena when winning the Committee Trophy at the Dublin Horse Show. The legendary Foxhunter had helped the British team to win a Bronze at the 1949 Olympic Games, and again in 1952, at Helsinki, when the team won the Gold. He died in November 1959 and his skeleton now stands at the Royal College of Veterinary Surgeons in London, alongside those of some of the great Derby winners. The legend of Foxhunter is still vividly remembered in the folklore of show-jumping.

Harry Llewellyn's team-mate in those days was Wilf White and his horse Nizefela, who raised excited cheers from the crowds each time they jumped. But it was not just for his big, accurate leaping that Nizefela had this effect on the public. It was his famous 'kick-back'. Each time he sailed over an obstacle he would kick-back his heels violently. He was in the team with Foxhunter that won the Gold medal at Helsinki, and in the Bronze-medal-winning squad at the 1956 Olympic Games. Horse and rider were one of the most consistent combinations on the international scene. Their performance was always reliable, and they became known as the 'fullback' of the British side. Wilf White was later awarded the OBE for his services to show-jumping.

Pat Smythe

But the rider who really caught the public's imagination in the 1950s was a modest and charming young girl who had jumped her way to the top on a shoestring budget. Patricia Rosemary Smythe became the idol of every horse-crazy schoolgirl in the world. She started in junior jumping before World War II but in the immediate post-war years she soon joined the ranks at the top of adult international jumping.

Her first famous horse was Finality, but others soon followed, such as Prince Hal, Tosca and Flanagan. On Prince Hal she cleared 2·25m (7ft 4½in) to win the Ladies' European High Jump record. Pat Smythe is the only lady rider to have won the European Championship four times. She was also the first female rider to compete at the Olympic Games. Riding Mr Robert Hanson's Flanagan, she was in the British squad at Stockholm in 1956 that won the Bronze; on the same mount she competed at the Rome Games in 1960. Pat's successes in the sport, including major wins at leading shows, international success in Nations' Cup teams, Grand Prix, Championships and the classic Queen Elizabeth II Cup for lady riders at the Royal International Horse Show when she rode Mr Pollard.

International Showjumping

It was not only in the England of the 1950s that

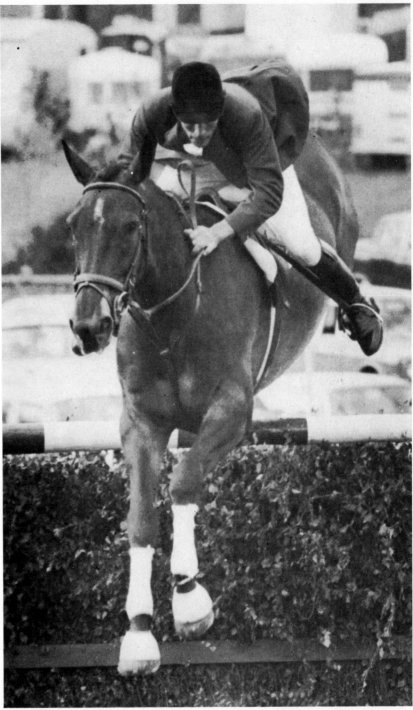

the popularity of show-jumping was gaining momentum. In America, Hugh Wiley and his brilliant horse Nautical were receiving much publicity and providing excitement for spectators. The American riders used the forward style of riding with grace. Freedom, the great American ideal, is the secret of their relaxed and easy style. Their horses are mostly thoroughbreds and usually have colourful names such as Nautical, Untouchable, Czar d'Esprit, Tomboy, Sinbad and Idle Dice. American riders like Hugh Wiley, Frank Chapot, Mary Mairs, Kathy Kusner, Bill Steinkraus and the talented professional, Rodney Jenkins, have become noted for the cool elegance, efficiency and simplicity of their riding.

Bill Steinkraus, one of America's most senior

Above *A popular combination in Britain, Paddy McMahon riding Pennwood Forge Mill. Although excluded from the 1972 Olympic team on the grounds of inexperience, they took the Men's European Championship in 1973.*

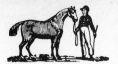

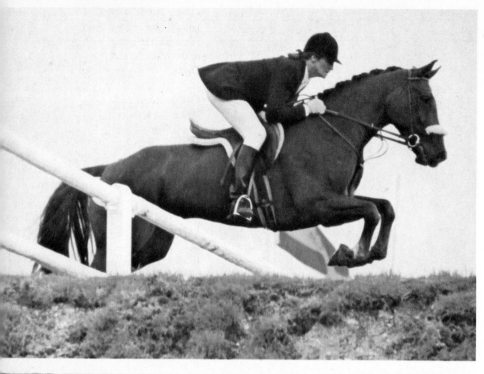

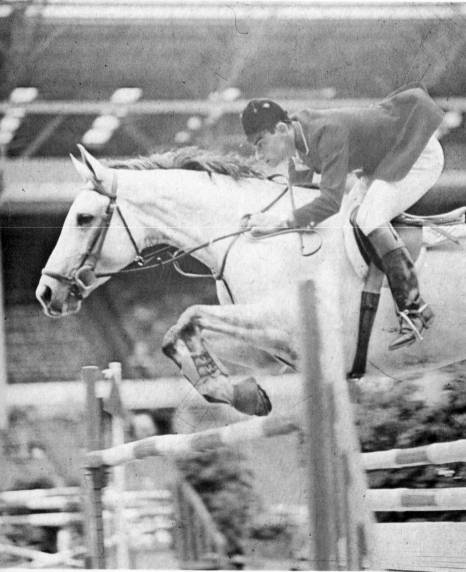

riders, left his horses alone as much as possible and then, at the vital moment, moved his body and hands gracefully to follow the parabola of his horse's flight over the fence, landing lightly on the other side to flow on to the next fence.

Alan Oliver

In England, the first of the television stars of show-jumping was Alan Oliver. Riding Red Admiral he became known to television viewers as a sort of equestrian dare-devil, willing to take risks and attempt very difficult jumps. At that time Alan and Red Admiral seemed to be the only English pair who could square-up to a nearly 7ft (2·1m) wall with the same gusto as the Americans and the Continentals.

Alan Oliver is the finest exponent of the physical school of riding. A natural gymnast, he defies all the rules of equitation with feet firmly planted in the irons, back rounded, and short, fixed reins. He is brilliant at presenting his horse to a fence, and never allows his horse to get into a gear that he has not asked for, or that he is not dictating. With martingale and bridle Alan has each horse controlled its energy concentrated and contained within the shortened form of its body. This he controls until he sees the right place to leave the ground and negotiate the obstacle. It is when the horse is in the air that Oliver's true genius as an athlete can be seen. By getting his weight off the horse's back Alan achieves the objective of giving his mount freedom in flight.

Red Admiral v The Rock

Red Admiral's great rival was The Rock. They jumped off against each other so often, especially at the White City, London, that it was not so much a battle, more of a double act. The Rock was ridden by Piero D'Inzeo, an Italian army officer. Where Alan Oliver was the athlete of his partnership, The Rock was the athlete in D'Inzeo's. A big, dapple grey, Irish-bred horse, it was well-made, full of quality and, through education, extremely supple. D'Inzeo epitomized the Italian school of natural equitation evolved over the centuries.

Hickstead

Some years ago, the first permanent show-jumping track in Britain was opened at the All England Jumping Course at Hickstead, Sussex. It is here that one of the major events in the international show-jumping calendar is staged: the All England Jumping Derby (similar to the Hamburg Derby), perhaps the severest and most testing show-jumping competition outside the Olympics. Riders come from Brazil, Germany, Australia, Italy, France, the United States and Ireland, in the hope of taking home this valuable prize. The show-jumper can be seen at his most exciting when tackling the massive and now world famous Hickstead Bank, one of the trickiest obstacles on this big, long and natural course. Hickstead provides all the excitement and tech-

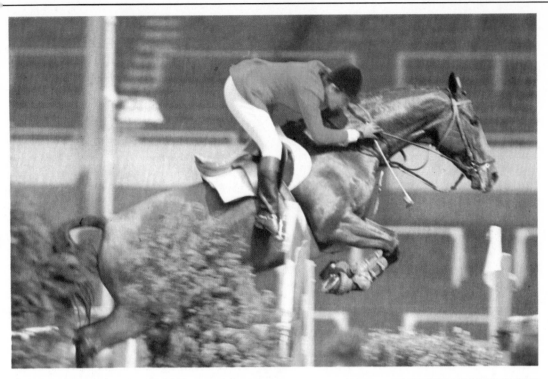

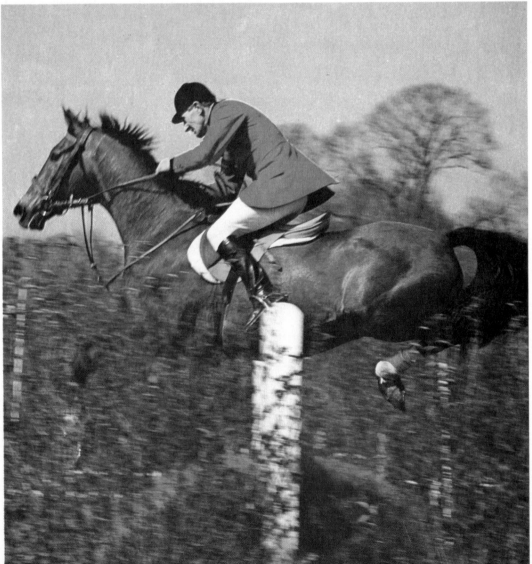

Opposite page above
Anneli Drummond-Hay on Xanthos, riding to victory in the 1969 British Jumping Derby.

Opposite page below
American showjumper Frank Chapot on Canadian Fall. In 1960 Chapot was a member of the United States team that won a silver medal at the Rome Olympics.

Left *Janou Tissot (neé Lefebvre) the reigning Women's World Champion. Since her marriage, however, she has been seen little on the world circuit.*

Below left *A veteran of the showjumping ring, Ted Williams who was still riding winners when younger members of the profession had retired.*

Below *Bill Steinkraus who took the first American equestrian Olympic Gold medal on Snowbound at Mexico.*

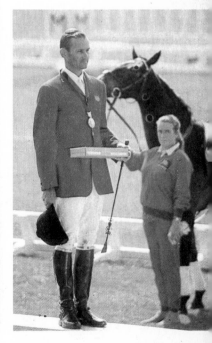

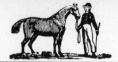

Right *The Australian John Fahey on Bonvale, the horse on which he so nearly gained a bronze medal in the 1964 Tokyo Olympics.*

Below right *Marion Mould on the incomparable Stroller. Although only 14.2 hands high, Stroller was ridden to victory in the 1970 Women's European Championships and took the silver medal in the 1968 Mexico Olympics.*

Opposite page *The reigning Men's World Champion, Hartwig Steenken, on Simond, his Hanoverian chestnut mare.*

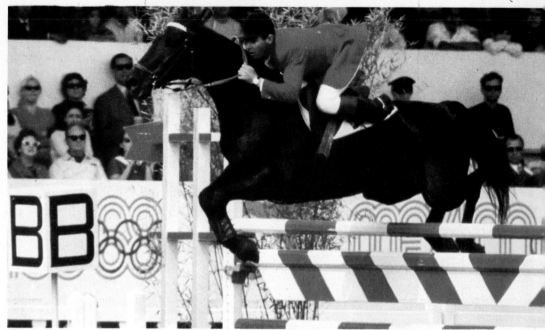

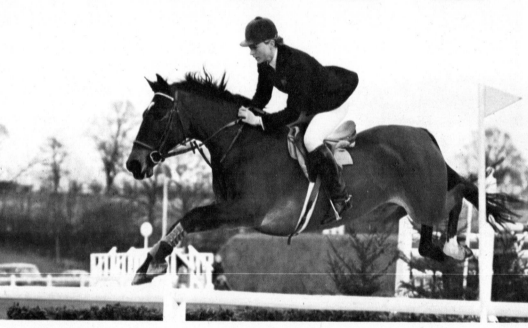

nical skills which are the traits of modern showing all over the world.

Today, international show-jumping is not far behind racing in popularity. The public flock to see great riders and horses, as the last decade has produced a crop of talented riders never before seen in the sport. From Britain these include Peter Robeson, Olympic medallist and classical horseman par excellence, Harvey Smith, perhaps the finest show-jumping rider the game has ever seen, David Broome, ex-world champion and the finest natural horseman in the world, as well as youngsters like Graham Fletcher, Roland Ferny-hough and Tony Newberry.

Recent international riders from France include gold medallist Pierre Jonquères d'Oriola and Jean-Michel Gaud. The leading Australian rider is John Fahey while in neighbouring New Zealand, John Cottle is considered a member of the art. Ireland possess the most exciting young rider on the scene, Eddie Macken. Germany, one of the most powerful jumping nations, has present World Champion Hartwig Steenken with his brilliant mare, Simona, the brothers Alwin and Paul Schockemohle, Hans Gunter Winkler, winner of a world championship, numerous Olympic medals and two King George V Gold Trophies; and the dashing and glamourous Hendrik Snoek. The new American riders include the red-headed Rodney Jenkins with his relaxed, flowing, but deadly accurate style. In Italy, the home of modern equitation, Graciano Mancinelli, an ex-world champion, is the leading rider. Well-known modern lady riders include Caroline Bradley, Olympic medallist Marion Mould and Judy Crago as well as America's diminutive ace Michele McEvoy, and present ladies world champion, Janou Tissot, from France.

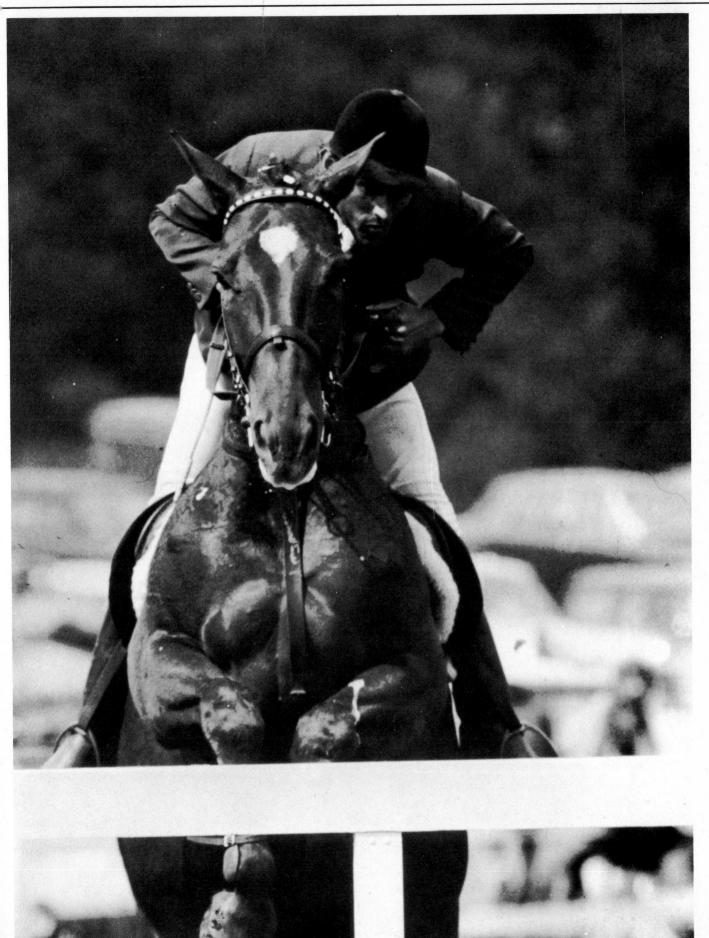

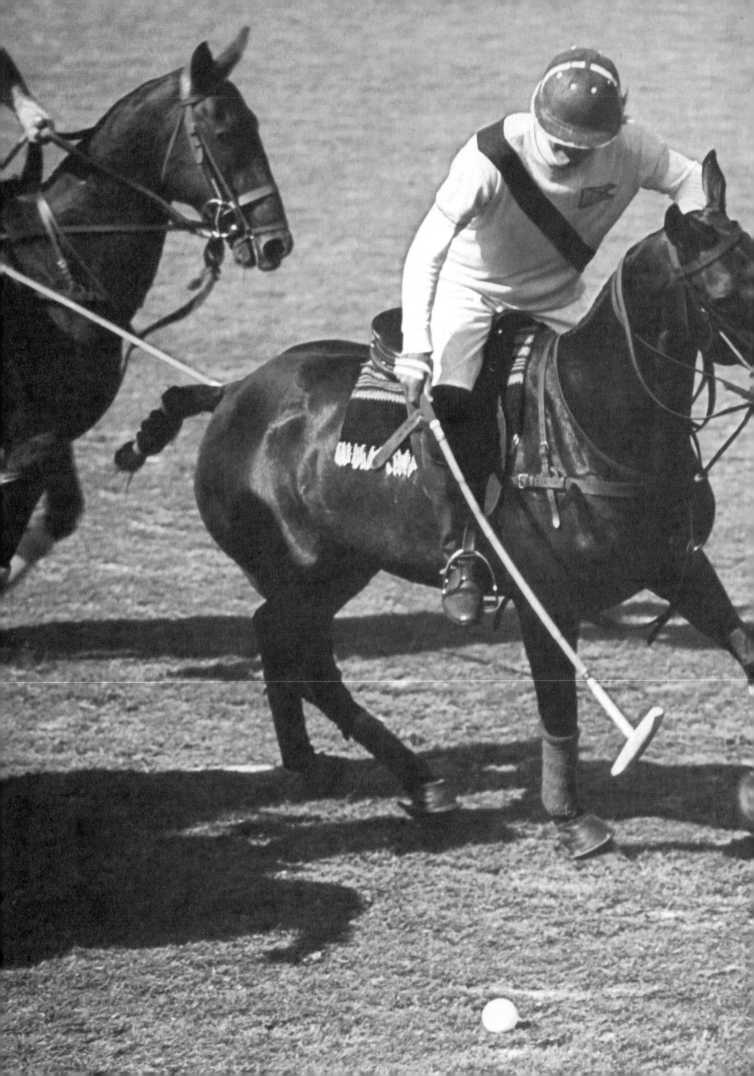

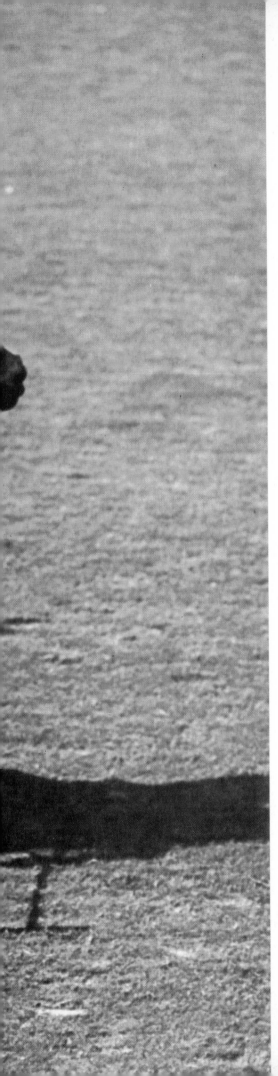

Polo -
Legacy from the Raj

The origins of Polo are lost in the mists of antiquity but there are records of similar games played in 525 BC. In Persia and in Assam at Manipuv, a game resembling lawn tennis was played on horses and called Chaugan. The game eventually took on a form nearer to polo. Historical records reveal that the first international played between the Iranians and Touranians caused a great stir and that during the reign of Chosroes II (628–591 BC) it was very popular as a ladies' game. There is not a great deal of difference between the game played then and the type of game played today in the big international tournaments in America and England. But it was not until the days of the British Raj that the game became popular in the West. British officers serving on the North-west frontier discovered the game and brought it back to England in 1869. In Assam, tea planters were playing it in 1850.

The development of the Polo pony

Some experts say that the 10th Hussars introduced the game into England on their return from India. The first public game was played at Hounslow in 1869. At that time not much thought was given to the type of pony used or to any specialized form of training. The emphasis tended to be on the skill of the player rather than on the training and ability of the pony. In the early days of polo a true pony was used with success. But it was not long before the Australian ponies proved themselves superior to the native ponies. In England, for example, small Irish horses were used. In Egypt, Sudan and India the Arab was ridden in the game. By 1914 the tough and wiry, Australian pony dominated top-class polo. This was especially true in India, which was considered to be the leading polo country of the world. In Britain, several leading polo players began to breed a special type of small hunter, which stood at 14.2 hands high. A Polo Pony Stud Book was started and the breed was based on native pony mares crossed with small thoroughbred stallions. But after the World War I this petered out and the breed, as such, disappeared.

By the early 1900s the sport was becoming a much more serious affair and international competition began to take the shape and form that is known today. In the England versus America match for the 1914 Meadowbrook Cup, which England won, the teams were mounted on English and American thoroughbreds. But with the coming of the World War I the sport went into a decline where, as far as England was concerned,

Lost largely in the mists of antiquity, the origins of polo can be traced back thousands of years before the British brought the game home and turned it into an international sport.

103

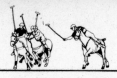

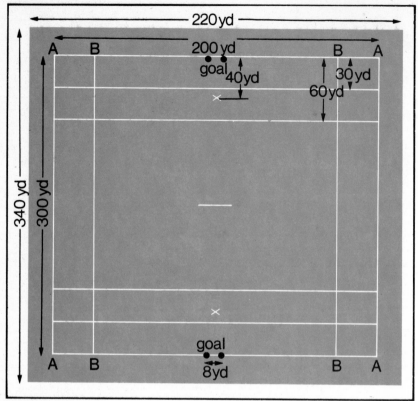

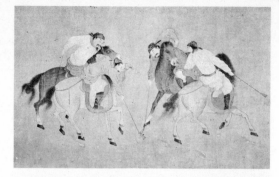

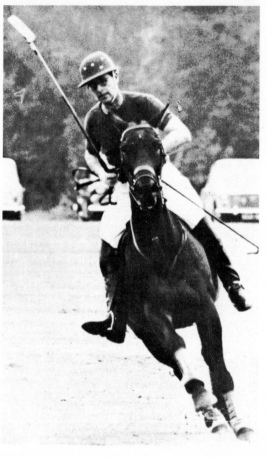

Above *A diagram of the field. The area between lines A and B is the safety zone, but it is not always indicated.*

Above right *The origins of the sport? Chinese players from a handscroll watercolour on silk from 1635 but probably based on an earlier original 1280-1386.*

Right *The Duke of Edinburgh was a keen competitor until his recent retirement from the game.*

it was to stay until relatively recent years. In America and the Argentine the sport remained strong.

From the ranches of the Argentine and Western America came the cow pony. It was found that he adapted well to the game but he was somewhat common in appearance and lacked a turn of foot. In second-class polo the cow pony became the standard type but the Argentinians, unaffected by war and realizing that they had the resources for cheap production, began creating a polo pony. This they did by importing thoroughbred blood and in-crossing it with the cow pony. By 1930, the Argentine pony was as good, if not better, than the English and American small thoroughbred pony. They now had the looks and speed, and had retained their original toughness and bone. In high-goal American Polo the Argentine pony has dominated the game since 1930.

Since 1947, the Argentine players have become the most powerful force in the sport and their ponies have been accepted as a separate breed. The breeding is very selective, using only mares which have proved themselves good at the game. In modern polo the 'pony power' of a team is 90 per cent of its success. For the players, their skill with stick and ball is obviously vital but it is their horsemanship that can really be the match winner.

Between the world wars the nursery for all the great British players was India. But since the late 1940s most of the best players have come from America and Argentina. The game started in America in 1883 and has grown both as an outdoor and an indoor sport. As in ancient times, it is played by women as well. Across the board of the equestrian sporting scene lady riders have

always competed on equal terms with the men, and in polo there are, and have been, some really fine lady players.

Nowadays, polo is very international and although very expensive, it does have a public following as a spectacle. The players no longer come from the ranks of the military and many of them are professionals. International seasons at Deauville, France, Smith's Lawn and Windsor, England, and in America and the Argentine comprise the game's calendar.

Rules and regulations

The rules are administered by the Hurlingham Club in England, the United States Polo Association and the Argentine Polo Association. There is no off-side rule in polo. The official handicap list is published by the Hurlingham Club for all players. The highest handicap a player can have is ten goals, and for teams, 40 goals is the maximum. A full size ground must not exceed 274m

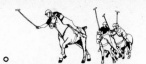

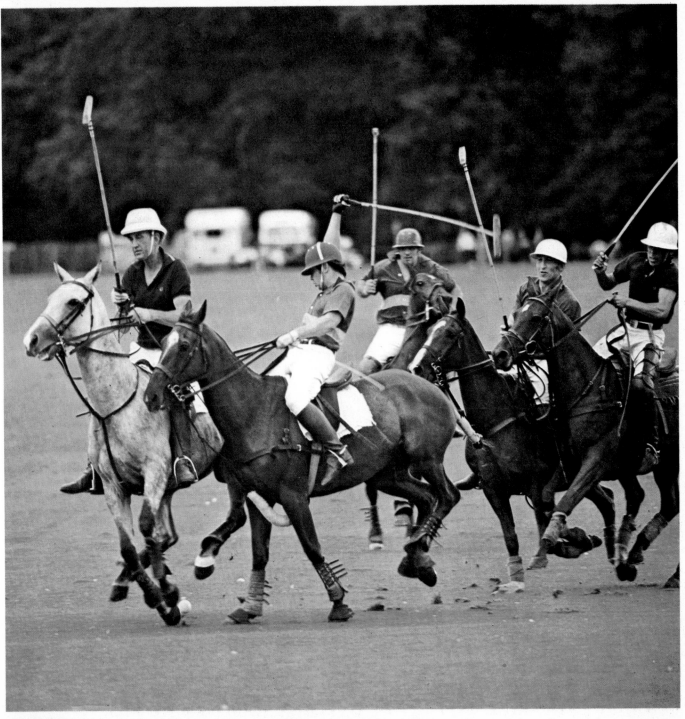

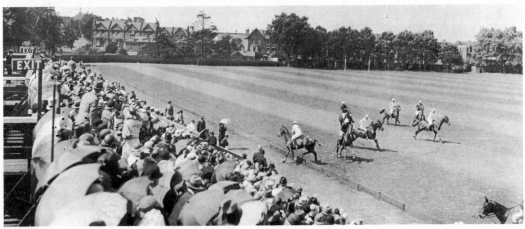

Above *The swinging of sticks and the congestion of the area will not daunt the truly trained polo pony. Trained to a high peak, he will never falter, and remain obedient and receptive on every occasion.*

Left *A match in progress, at Hurlingham, one of the early centres of English polo.*

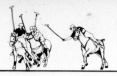

Right *Leaning out to take the shot. The successful polo player is not necessarily a brilliant horseman but is usually a natural ball-player.*

Below *Polo has been a popular sport in Australia for three generations. The game is played mainly by pastoralists and during important carnivals, which extend over three or four days, players and spectators travel hundreds of miles to the matches.*

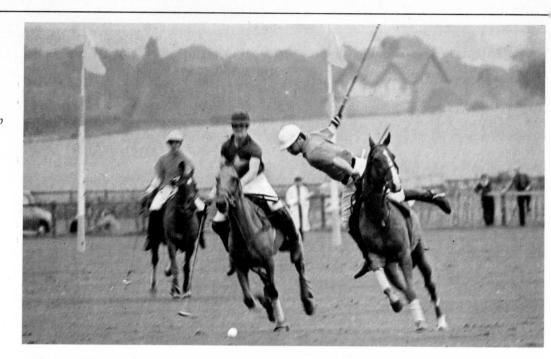

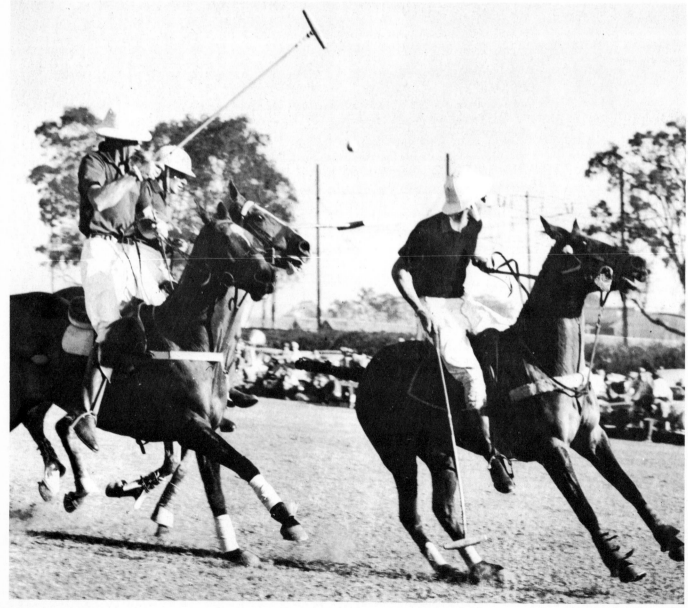

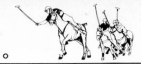

(300yd) in length, by 183m (200yd) in width (if unboarded), and 274m (300yd) in length and 146m (160yd) in width if boarded. The surface of the playing area may be grass, dirt or tan.

The polo ball used must not exceed 83mm (3·25in) in diameter and its weight must be within the range 128–142gm (4·5–5oz). A match ball is made of willow and bamboo and a practice ball is made of foam rubber. The polo stick is some 1·3m (51in) in length and is generally made of malacca. The head of the stick is made from bamboo root but other light, tough woods may be used, such as persimmon. There is no official definition of the stick's size and shape.

The number of players in a polo match is limited to four aside in all matches and games. These make a formation of three up front and one back. The game is played in seven periods, or chukkas, of 8min each (in the United States eight periods of 7½min). The umpires, usually two, are mounted. A referee and a goal judge control the game and a goal is scored when the ball is hit between the posts and across the goal line. The rules tend to vary slightly from country to country but these are the simple basic regulations. While easy to follow they are framed to reduce the danger as much as possible.

Polo players travel around the world circuits with teams of ponies. Large audiences are attracted. The crowds can be brought to their feet by star performers as they gallop flat-out down the boards of the long side of the pitch, their agile ponies shouldering-off an opponent, to drive home a winning goal. In England, leading players like Paul Withers, The Duke of Edinburgh, Prince Charles and show-business personality Jimmy Edwards, or men like the American Roy Barry are the leading lights and the crowd-pullers. But for the spectators it is the tough little horses of dainty feet and swift action who provide a great source of entertainment. They sometimes seem to know more about the game than their reinsmen and their competitive spirit urges them on to follow the action and the ball.

Below *HRH Prince Charles mounted on a superb grey polo pony during a game in Malta.*

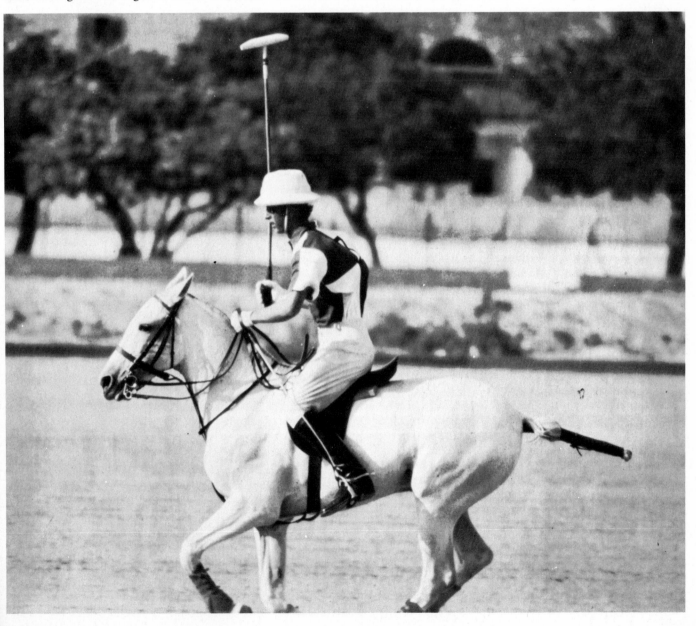

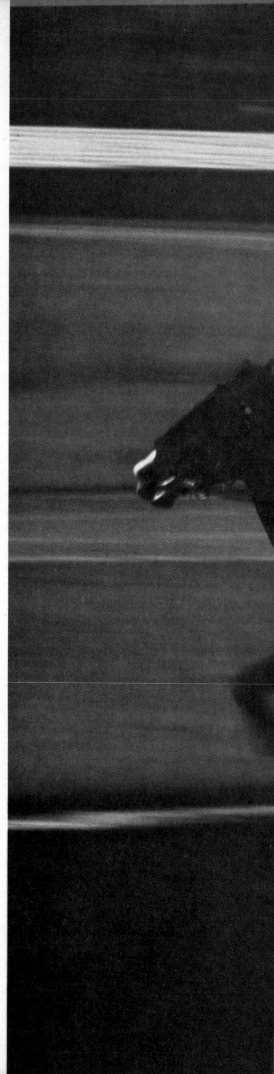

Trotting & Pacing

The sport of trotting horses originated from the ancient Egyptians, Greeks and Romans. Chariot-racing, the forerunner of this exciting sport, was an everyday happening. When not out warring or hunting, horses and chariots would be taken to the local arena for a day's racing. These affairs were fairly rough, competition was fierce and it was not unusual for horses and drivers to be involved in dramatic crashes and fatal accidents. But with the passing of time the chariot developed into a vehicle of transportation and haulage, and with the coming of heavier wagons a stronger and less agile horse was used in harness.

Ambling

It was in rural England, in pre-mechanized days, that the sport reappeared and once again the crowds flocked to country fairs to see the trotting races. The light carriage was a common sight on the unmade, bumpy roads of that time. Tradesmen, small businessmen and farmers all kept fine framed horses, as against heavy horses, in the same way that the average modern family keeps a car. These horses were used for business and communications. And competition soon crept in as a diversion. The Ambler became known as a type of driving horse.

Ambling is a gait created by man and totally unnatural to the horse. The harness horse was trained to simultaneously raise and lower his hind-legs and fore-legs on one side of his body. For example, near-fore and near-hind would move together, and then off-fore and off-hind would make the next stride. The horse's body was put out of balance by this and also took considerably more strain than in the natural trot. But the end product, although tiring for the horse, was a gait that was smooth and gliding in action as well as being very fast. It was very popular, particularly, in the East of England, which was the home of early trotting and ambling racing.

Trotters and pacers

There are two types of trotter—the pacer and the trotter. It is from the Ambler that pacing came. The horse is trained to race with a lateral action known as pacing. The trotter, in contrast, is trained to race at an extended version of the natural trot. In other words, his limbs move in the normal diagonal sequence, off-fore with near-hind, and near-fore with off-hind.

Trotting is to racing what show-jumping is to equestrianism—a sport of the people. The people

Although the competitor faces elimination if his horse breaks into a canter, the well-trained trotter can achieve great speeds by racing at an extended version of his natural trot.

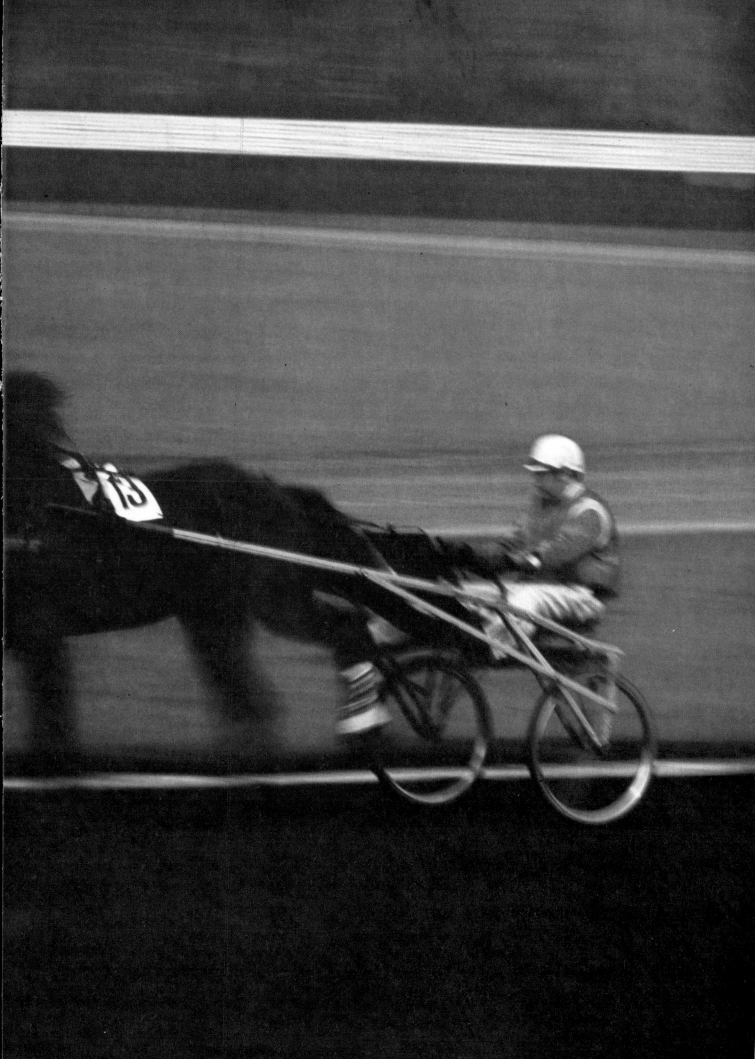

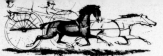

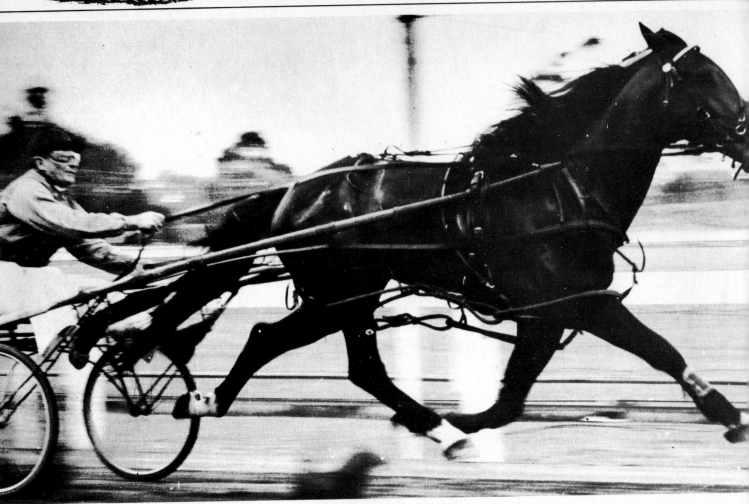

Above *Pacing is one of the most popular sports in Australia. Here pacer James Scott, who took the Inter-Dominion Pacing Championship in 1962, guided by P. Hall. A win in a major competition such as this can often lead to lucrative offers to race in the United States.*

Opposite page bottom right *Americans are often keen to buy Australian stock, mainly for breeding purposes. In 1969 a record sum was paid for this horse Adaptor, winner of the Miracle Mile.*

Opposite page bottom left *The pacer is often hoppled, an invention dating from Elizabethan times to prevent a lady's horse from galloping off.*

involved were neither aristocracy nor rich industrialists. Racing, the 'Sport of Kings', was labelled the pastime of the devil by puritanical regimes and stories of scandals, betting swindles and corruption tended to give a touch of reality to this image, an image which still exists for many today. In fact, in some states in 19th-century America, thoroughbred breeding and racing was banned or suspended for a period. But trotting has never suffered from the turmoil caused by reformers or guardians of the public morality. But for many racing men, trotting never has been and never will be accepted as 'real' racing.

Organized flat-racing and steeplechasing took over completely from trotting in England. The sport almost totally disappeared and has never been popular again. But in America, Canada and Australia, the settlers soon established harness racing and its popularity has gone from strength to strength.

Many of the famous Norfolk trotters were exported and became the foundation stock of the American trotters and pacers. Many of these Norfolk and Lincoln trotters and pacers found their way to New England and it was from these that the roadster strains now used in America were born. They were of the saddle-horse type but with a smooth gait and willing temperament which made them ideal for racing between the traces. The first of these strains were known as

Canadian and Narragansett pacers. So from these roots emerged the North American harness-racer.

The Standardbred

Organized breeding and well-known sires were soon established and great families such as the Copperbottoms and the Hyatogas were renowned for their swift horses. These families and other early star performers of the American Morgan breed were the foundation-line for the Standardbred. The Standardbred is now recognized as a breed and is one of the most successful bloodlines in the trotting game. In 1849 the breed was injected with thoroughbred blood through a horse called Hambletonian 10 which was also known as Rydsyk's Hambletonian. On his male and female line he traced back to an imported thoroughbred stallion, Messenger, and this sire is thought to have played an important part in creating the Standardbred. Many of the mares mated with Messenger were from non-blood lines and from this mixture of warm-blood (thoroughbred) and cold-blood (non-thoroughbred) evolved a type of horse with a natural flair for trotting.

The Standardbred relates to trotting and pacing in the way that the thoroughbred relates to racing, the only difference being that the non-Standardbred is allowed to race against his better-bred brothers and sisters but must be declared

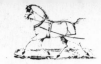

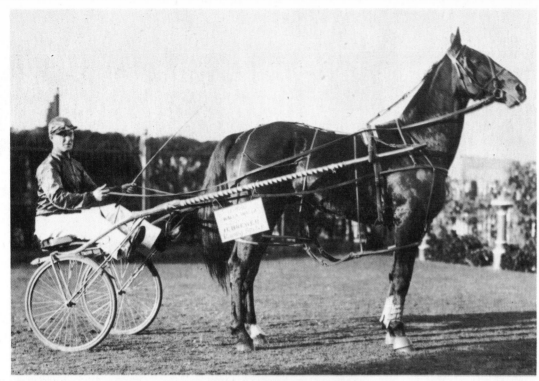

Left *One of Australia's greatest ever pacers, Walla Walla was so heavily handicapped that the phrase 'further back than Walla Walla' was coined to indicate an apparently hopeless position.*

Below left *Horses from New Zealand often participate in the Australian races. Here Caduceus takes the Inter-Dominion Pacing Championships*

Below *Chariot racing is often considered to be the forerunner of pacing. Here a design from a Greek water jar shows the horses being prepared for the race.*

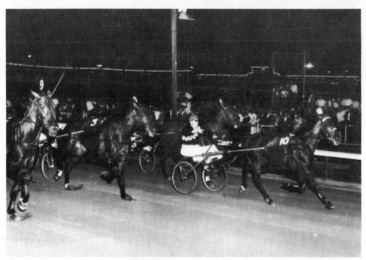

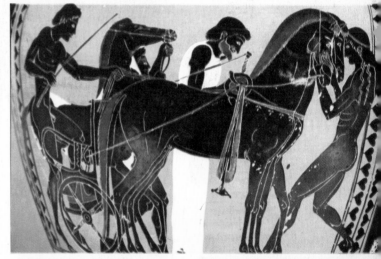

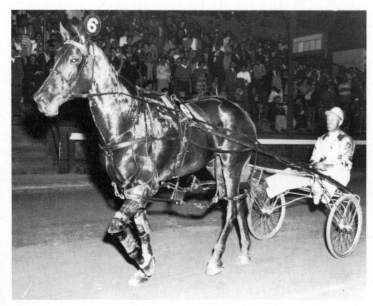

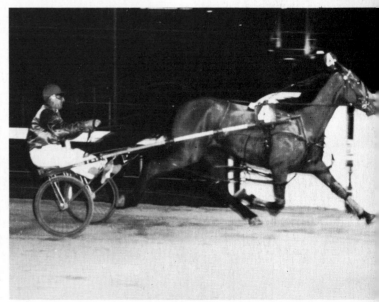

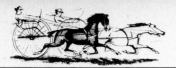

as a non-Standardbred, whereas in flat-racing the conditions are framed to exclude the non-thoroughbred. On the trotting-race programme this information would be given to the race fan, but in the modern sport the non-Standardbred is very rarely seen on the raceways.

The idea of calling the breed Standardbred was based, not on some purist theory of lineage but on a much more practical point of view. In the old days of trotting, a harness-horse was tested over a mile to see if he could cover it in what was accepted to be a standard time. If he passed this test then he was allowed to race in public. Today, the standard is fixed at 2 min 20 sec for 1 mile (1·6km). In modern trotting terms, this is not such a fantastic speed as it may at first seem. The raceways are now designed to encourage speeds similar to those seen on the flat-race tracks. Many of the race strips are 'blanked', automatic starting is in use and the modern sulky or carriage is light.

Harness-racing in America is older than the Republic itself and it thrived until the arrival of the motor car. With the horseless carriage taking over where the gig left off, less people owned or bred horses for racing between the traces. But by 1940 the sport began to regain its popularity. With the invention of the automated starting gate, the scheduling of night-time racing and the forming of the Pari-Mutual tote-betting system, the sport became more and more popular. Great racing stadiums with panoramic restaurants and facilities that the early settlers could never have imagined are now part of the sport's exciting scene. There are raceways like Roosevelt Park in the United States or Vincennes in Paris, with their floodlit cinder tracks drawing enormous crowds. The trotter and the Standardbred are no longer the poor relation of the thoroughbred but fill an important gap in the horse-orientated sector of the leisure solidus entertainment industry which is now so much a part of modern life.

The French trotter

Some one hundred years after the Americans had begun to develop the Standardbred, French coach-horse breeders, backed by the national stud, decided to do the same and used their own stock to create a trotting horse. The Norman horse used by the French was an all-purpose creature suitable for hunting, carting or agricultural work but during Napoleon's campaigns through sometimes accidental breeding, it picked up a sprinkling of Arab blood. After this era French tastes underwent a swing to everything English. Thoroughbreds, fashion, life-styles and furniture of English origin were passionately sought after. The French breeders imported non-thoroughbred hunters to cross with the Norman horse. The most famous of these was Young Rattler, a sire said to be found in the pedigree of every French trotter.

In modern times the French trotter has become more protected by the breed society and although

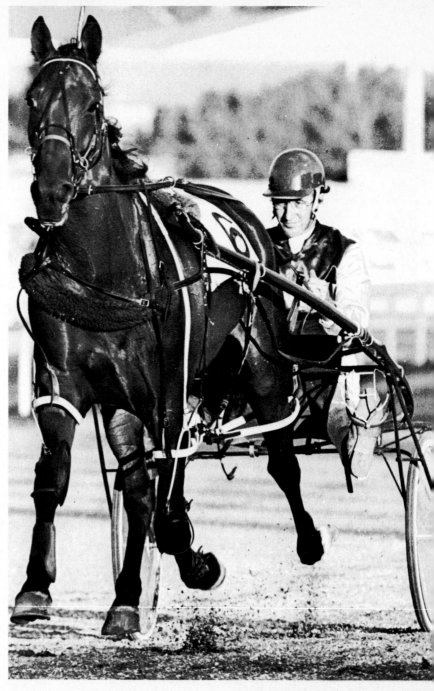

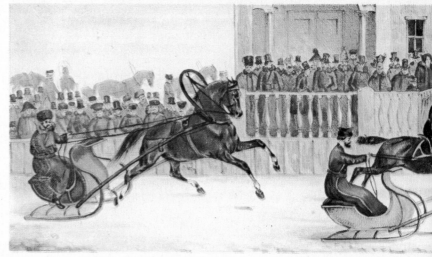

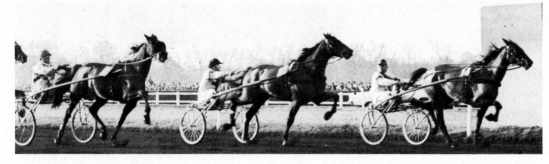

not a horse of great quality he is recognized as one of the best trotting strains throughout the world. The conditions are similar to those used in America for the Standardbred. The trotter must first prove he can cover 1km (0·6 mile) in 1 min 42sec in a public race. In 1942 the stud book was closed to any horse that could not be shown to have a registered sire and dam. So the French trotter was established in his own right.

Since then there have been several notable examples of the ability of the French horses. Jasmin, a pure-bred French trotter that went to the United States in the late 1950s, beat all the American leading Standardbreds at the fast Roosevelt Raceway. More recently, Roquepine thrilled the American race fans when making an all-conquering tour of the trotting tracks in

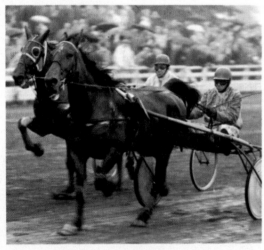

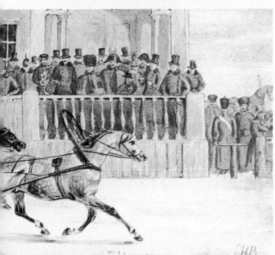

America. This French mare was almost unbeatable and is said to be the greatest trotter ever. She won all the important trotting races in America and on the Continent.

Trotting in Russia

In Russia, trotting is more popular than flat-racing. Much of this is due to an 18th-century breeder, Count Alexi Orlov. At his Khrenov stud in 1778, he experimented with the idea of a native harness-racer. Using an Arabian-descended stallion called Polkan and a Dutch mare, he set out to create a perfect trotter. In the year 1784 he produced a grey stallion which he christened Bars I. It was said of this celebrated horse that he had fine qualities and an outstanding action at the trot. He in turn was mated with cross-bred Arabian-Dutch mares and eventually through inbreeding and inheritance the Orlov trotter became accepted as a breed.

By the 19th century the Orlovs were one of the most famous breeds in Russia, and were kept almost exclusively for the racetrack. Through a methodical system of tests on racecourses the breed was improved. The first trotting races in Moscow had been held in 1799, and because of its popularity the evolution of the sport and the trotter is as well documented as the founding of the English thoroughbred. The Moscow Trotting Society was formed in 1834.

The tremendous improvements made in the Orlov trotter can be seen in the records. In 1836, the champion Bychok raced 3·2km (2 miles) in 5min 45sec. Then in 1866, Poteshny sped over the same distance in 5min 8sec. By the late 1800s, this time was reduced to 4min 46sec—proof that careful and selective breeding does increase performance.

The Orlov is not the only harness-racing breed to achieve success on the Russian tracks. The Russian trotter, which is the product of a long-term programme of selective crossing of the Orlov and imported American trotters, plays a competitive part in the sport. Smaller in stature than the Orlov he is nevertheless the faster of the two. The Russian trotter holds many national records, like the 1600 metres (nearly 1 mile) in 1min 59·6sec; 3·2km (2 miles) in 4min 10·4sec and the 6·4km (4 miles) in 8min 55sec. Race-meetings are staged at Moscow, Odessa, Kharkov, Kuibyshev, Perm and Alma-Ata race tracks, and in the winter months the drivers are carried on light sleighs.

Rodeo-
testing the traditional skills of the cowboy

Rodeo is a magic word that conjures up the spirit of early America. It incorporates the pioneering spirit of its founding fathers and the freedom of its vast plains, great land masses where wild horses roamed and men carved out new communities. Men who lived for, lived off and lived with the animal kingdom, the horse their companion and working partner, and the herding of beef steer their way of life and livelihood.

Cowboys and gauchos

The word rodeo comes from the Spanish 'rodear' meaning 'to go round'. The gauchos and the cowboys worked in small teams, guarding the herds and driving them each season to the large city stock markets. Their lives revolved around tending the young and the sick and training the wild animals. The prairies and the pampas were well stocked with mustangs, brought to this ancestral home of the horse by the Spanish conquistadores. The cow-pony was the lifeline of the man who worked on the range, with herds of mustang, criollo, pintos and palominos running alongside the cattle. If a cowboy or gaucho needed a horse all he had to do was to catch one.

The everyday life of the gauchos and cowboys

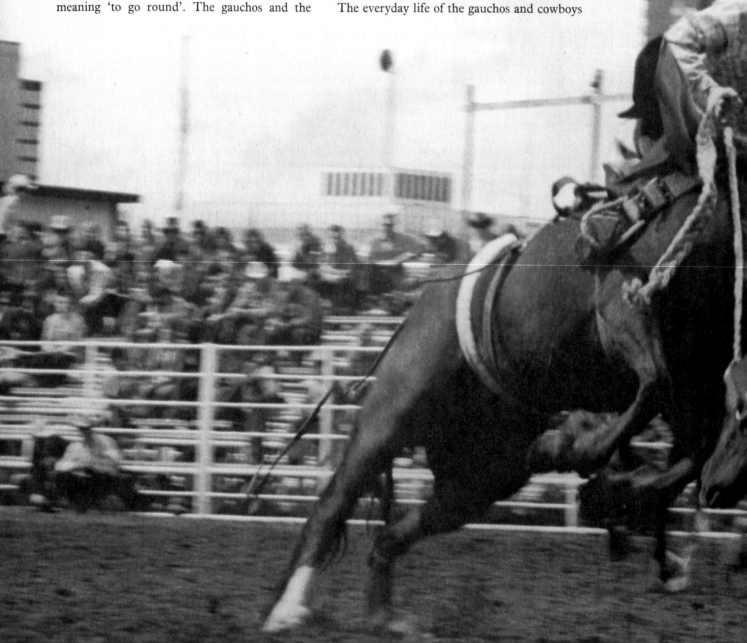

was involved in rounding up cattle, driving herds of horses and breaking in new ones for their work. Life was hard and it was lonely, out on the range for months on end. At night the camp fire illuminated the lean faces of the men of the prairie. Some would sing songs, telling the tale of untameable stallions or legendary drives along

Past are the days when bronc-busting or steer roping would form part of the cowboy's daily routine but such is the excitement of the spectacle that it lives on purely as a spectator sport.

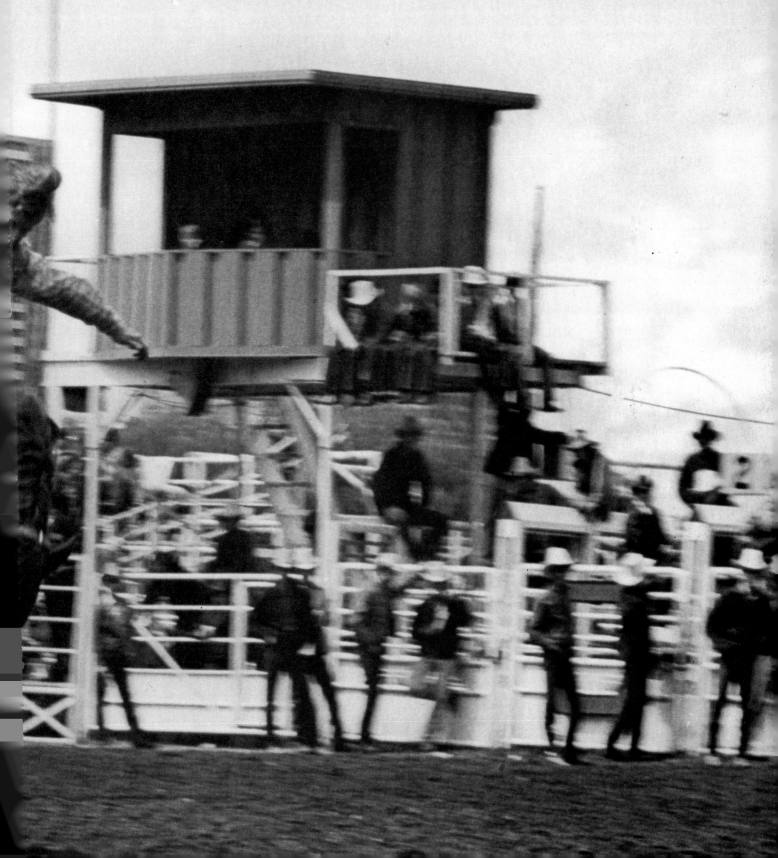

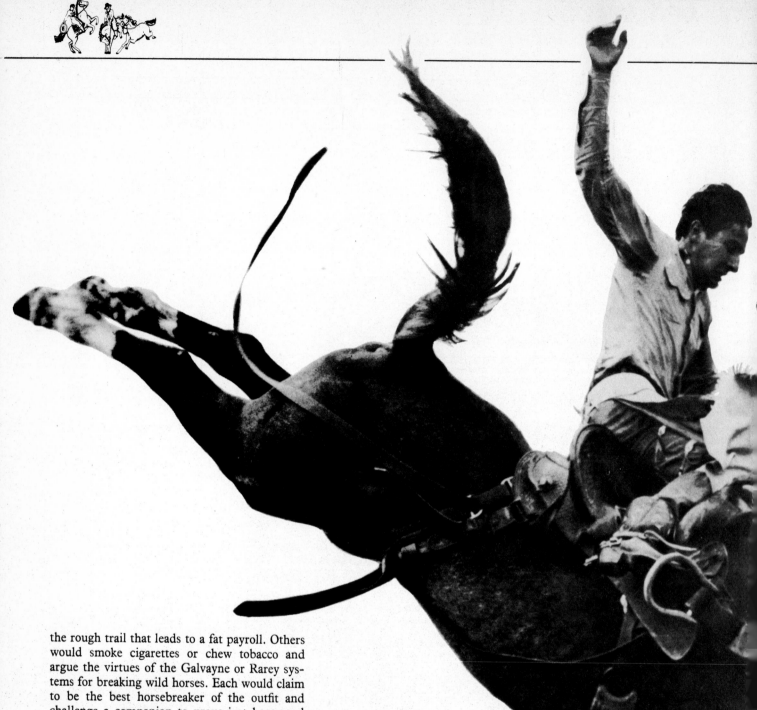

the rough trail that leads to a fat payroll. Others would smoke cigarettes or chew tobacco and argue the virtues of the Galvayne or Rarey systems for breaking wild horses. Each would claim to be the best horsebreaker of the outfit and challenge a companion to prove just how good he was. Man's inexplicable need to master the animal kingdom and to show himself superior to his colleagues soon turned into a competition event.

Sydney Galvayne was a celebrated, 19th-century horsebreaker and trainer. His theory was to use scientifically the great strength of the horse against itself and he boasted of never having a failure through his hands. He visited England in 1884 to lecture on his techniques, and in 1887 appeared before Queen Victoria.

John Solomon Rarey (1827–1866) was a farmer and horse tamer from Ohio. His method was to exhaust the horse before starting to work him or retrain him. Although the Rarey System is the better known of the two, the Galvayne method is generally accepted as being the more humane.

The rodeo as entertainment

The state fair became popular in America in the 18th and 19th centuries. Bronco-busting was part of the festival and the public loved it. The rodeo was born and was here to stay. But as the cowboy sauntered into the 20th century, the horse was relegated from his number one position on the range. The jeep and the estate wagon, with their radio telephones, took over. Above, the helicopter wheeled, watching over the grazing herds with an all-seeing eye.

The rodeo, along with the Hollywood-created cowboy, joined the commercial ranks of the entertainment industry. The great Western spectacle, based on the earlier daily life of the cowboy, is a big crowd-puller throughout the United States along the Pacific seaboard and into Canada. The new cowboy travels from one arena to another, and earns his living by showing his talent and prowess as a horseman to spectators, only

Main picture *Despite their rough condition, Broncs are usually in top condition and rarely become dispirited. Usually their ages range between 12 and 15 years.*

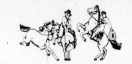

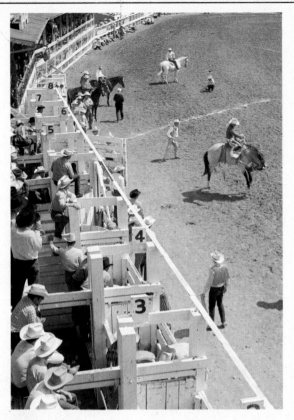

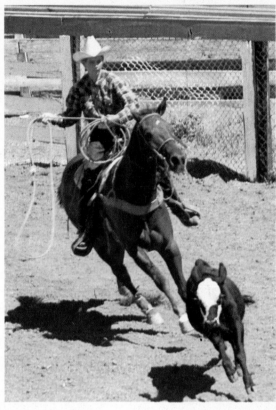

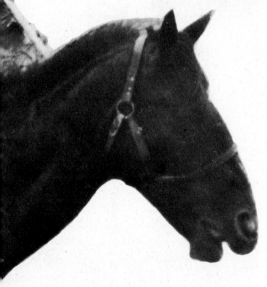

leaving the circuit from time to time for an enforced sojourn in the local hospital.

The programme of the rodeo is a demonstration of the skills the good cowboy should have, involving the roping of a steer or galloping after a steer, then leaping from his horse and catching the running animal by the horns and throwing him to the ground. Mastering the broncos and driving a team of four, spirited horses and open wagon in a winner-takes-all race are two more popular events. Riding wild bulls renowned for 'emptying' their rider and then in rage attacking him as he lies on the ground, is one of the more dangerous events. Rodeos also have a competition to find the champion roper. He must be able to lasso his steer, tie him to the horn of his Western saddle, dismount and throw his steer to the ground—all in less than ten seconds.

The most popular and most exciting attraction of the rodeo is the bronco-riding. The wild horse is brought into the chute without a saddle or bridle, just a webbing surcingle for the rider to hang on to. The cowboy climbs over the planking and on to the bony back of the bronc. He readies himself, getting a good grip on the surcingle. The rules state that he must keep one hand above his shoulder-line, and to be the champion of champions he must stay on the wild animal for more than ten seconds. He knows that as yet nobody has stayed there longer than seven seconds.

The barrier is opened and man and beast plunge into the arena amid roars from the crowd. The bronc starts buckjumping, trying to unseat his unwelcome rider by arching his back like a spring and jumping into the air with all four legs at once. The movement is fast and violent. The

Above left *The classic rodeo event. The rider must maintain his seat for 10 seconds using only his one rein hand.*

Above *In calf roping, the rider must rope the calf, dismount and throw it and then cross and tie any three legs.*

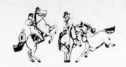

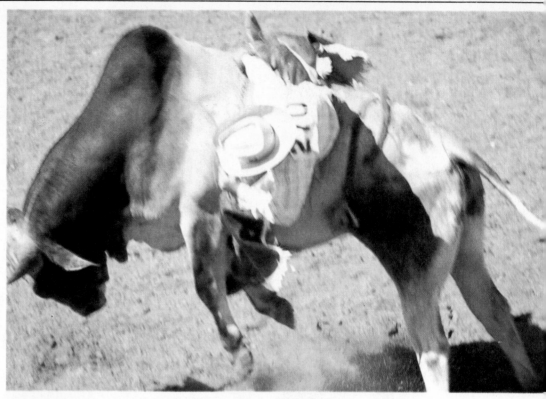

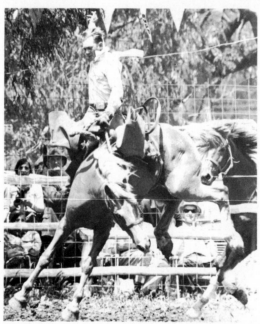

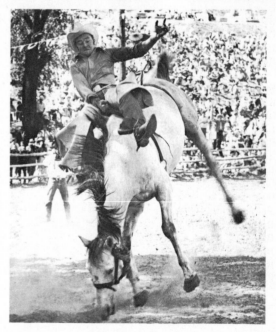

cowboy sways backwards and forwards to the movement, trying to keep his balance by using his legs. With each buckjump or pig-jump, where the bronc is leaping and kicking at the same time, his position gets less and less secure. In barely six seconds, which feel like a lifetime for the rider, the ground comes rushing at him and the panting bronco swerves away from the man in the dust, lashing out with his hind-legs.

The stars of the rodeo spectacle become celebrities in their own right. Everybody knows the masters of the bucking-broncos and the virtuosi of the lasso. At the famous Calgary Stampede in Canada, the mad race of the chuck-wagons is the show-stopper. The driver has four horses to handle, as his wagon bumps and sways round the racecourse. Driver and horses give their maximum, as if the race to the line were not for a prize but for the richest gold stake. Sometimes, in the hustling of the race, the trace-harness breaks but the horses still continue to pull the chuck-wagon by the reins only, to cross the line at break-neck speed.

In the smaller town, the rodeo is still the true traditional festival, where local cattlemen and horse breeders gather together in joyous reunion for several hectic and unforgettable days. Nationwide, the rodeo, with a long and romantic heritage, is now America's second-largest equestrian spectator sport, after flat-racing.

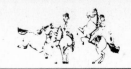

Index

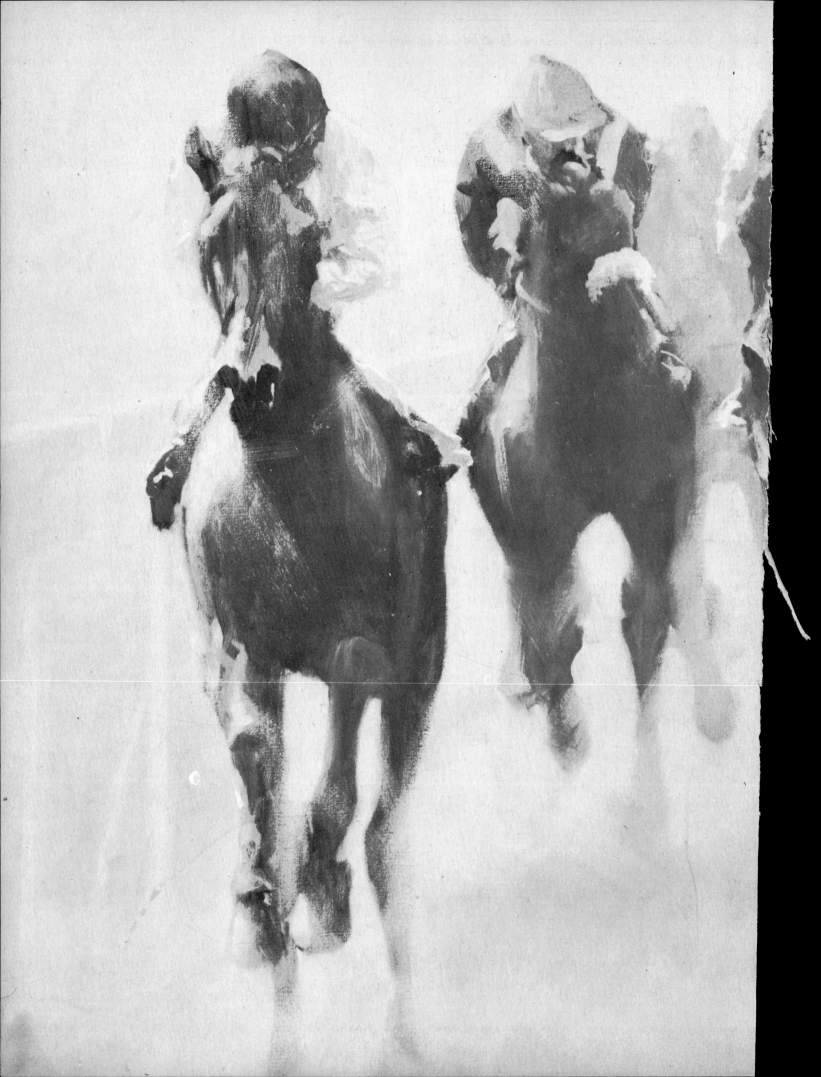